Surviving

Alzheimer's

Practical tips and soul-saving wisdom

for caregivers

PAULA SPENCER SCOTT

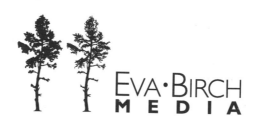

EVA·BIRCH
MEDIA

For Dad, Gram, Louie, and Emily,

and all those we miss due to dementia

PRAISE FOR *SURVIVING ALZHEIMER'S*

"Knowledge is power in the fight against memory loss and Alzheimer's Disease. In *Surviving Alzheimer's*, Paula Spencer Scott combines her years of experience with information-packed, easy-to-read — and most important, truly meaningful — words of wisdom from herself as well as countless experts. This is a must-read for anyone impacted by the stress of caring for someone with Alzheimer's."

— *Richard Isaacson, MD, director of the Alzheimer's Disease Prevention & Treatment Program, Weill Cornell Medical College / New York Presbyterian Hospital and co-author,* The Alzheimer's Diet

"Regular doses of Paula Spencer Scott's supportive and instructive wisdom should be prescribed to every family member dealing with Alzheimer's. Her why-this, try-this approach is a winner. It's like a first-aid kit for stressed family caregivers."

— *Lisa P. Gwyther, MSW, LCSW, associate professor, Duke University School of Medicine; director, Duke Family Support Program, and co-author,* The Alzheimer's Action Plan

"Fantastic!"

— *Leeza Gibbons, co-host of "America Now" and founder of the Leeza Gibbons Memory Foundation*

"Terrific and highly recommended"

— *Alzheimer's Prevention and Treatment News, February 2014*

"**Paula Spencer Scott has a gift;** she is one of the rare people who is able to write about complex medical topics and make them interesting and clear. In this book, she takes on one of the quiet crises of our time, the increasing number of people who are doing all they can to care for someone with dementia. All dementia caregivers need help. This book is a wonderful gift to the millions of families on the dementia-care treadmill. If you know one of these heroes, or if you're a caregiver yourself — run, don't walk, to order it!"

— *Kenneth Robbins, MD, MPH, clinical professor of psychiatry, University of Wisconsin, and geriatric psychiatrist*

"**Insightful and practical guidance** for the millions of caregivers struggling to help their loved ones suffering from dementia."

— *Gary Small, MD, director of the UCLA Longevity Center and co-author,* The Alzheimer's Prevention Program

"**A treasure trove of practical information,** addressing so many of the real-world questions and problems that I see dementia caregivers struggle with every day. This is a well-researched book that synthesizes the knowledge and experiences of a diverse group of experts (not the least of which is Paula herself) into clear explanations and actionable advice. A great choice to recommend to patients and families."

— *Leslie Kernisan, MD, MPH, geriatrician and caregiver educator, University of California, San Francisco*

"Surviving Alzheimer's **is full of good advice and helpful hints.** I am so glad that there is real help now for families who are on the journey of dementia with loved ones. "

— *Virginia Bell, MSW, creator, The Best Friends Approach to Alzheimer's Care and "The Alzheimer's Disease Bill of Rights"*

WHY I WROTE THIS BOOK

When the first shoe dropped, I wasn't yet thinking about Alzheimer's — at least, not in a personal sense.

At the time, I was editing the Alzheimer's channel for what was then a new website, Caring.com. My specialties as a journalist have always been health, family, and women's concerns. I've co-authored five books with doctors, been a columnist for two national magazines, and written countless articles on these subjects. So the site's mission — to provide family caregivers with support and eldercare information — appealed to my longtime interests in an academic and professional way.

That was in 2007, and at the time, I had two relatively healthy parents.

Or so I thought.

It's about my parents

"I just thought you should know," my mom called to say, in the same casual tone she usually said things like, *How are the kids?* and *I got a good deal on yarn today,* "that I fell and broke my pelvis and pubic bone." Since I was cooking dinner and helping a child with homework while juggling the phone, I wasn't quite sure I'd heard right.

"You don't really need to come up," she added. That was momspeak for, *Help!* My parents were in their early 80s. Of course I went up, from where I lived in North Carolina back to my childhood home in suburban Detroit. My brother, Paul, also came up from North Carolina to help. (The other three siblings, in three different states, would take later shifts, not that we yet realized a need for it.)

It took a day for us to set up a temporary downstairs bedroom in which Mom could recuperate.

It took half a day for the other shoe to drop — discovering the extent to which she'd been covering for Dad.

Sure, his memory had been a little spacey lately. But he'd always had a bit of the goofy, absent-minded professor in him. Though he'd been moving more slowly, he still golfed and bowled — longest-continuous member of his General Motors bowling league, since 1948. He still sent us all snapshots of his tomatoes and hibiscus flowers that he'd printed himself, didn't he? Big travelers, our parents liked to make road trips from one child's home to the next. Sure, the videos Dad had begun taking of the passing highway, mile after uneventful mile, while Mom drove, might have been a sign something was up. But he was just getting older, right?

So we told ourselves.

It's one thing to see someone with cognitive trouble for a few days as a guest in your home or at quick, chaotic family celebrations. Actually living with him in his home is a whole other plane of reality check. When Paul and I arrived, the dryer was clanking so angrily that he went straight to the basement to investigate. "Oh, it's just gotten loud," said Mom. (Paul found black oil pooled beneath it.) Calling home to say I'd arrived, the connection kept shorting out. (Paul later discovered a wiring problem.) Minutes later, I punched 2:00 into the microwave to heat water for tea; the machine worked, but the number display didn't. All these were unthinkable lapses for Dad, a former mechanical engineer who was such a home-repair geek that I didn't realize until my 20s that professional plumbers and electricians even existed.

And that was just the first half hour. Heating up dinner, I noticed a huge grease fire under a stove burner. ("Oh, your dad was making soup and got distracted.") The next morning, Dad seemed surprised to see me: "When did you get here? Are you in town on business?"

That was a Sunday. We took him to church. "How nice to see you! Where's Eleanore?" asked my mom's best friend.

"Oh, she hurt her side and she can't walk too good," Dad told her.

"Um, she broke her pelvis and she can hardly walk at all," I clarified.

I began to learn how many meaningful conversations you can have with your siblings just by meeting gazes and raising eyebrows.

Dad forgot his standing Monday golf game. His old buddy Bob pulled me aside when he came to pick him up, while waiting for him to get ready. "He's getting worse, isn't he?" he said, tapping his forehead meaningfully.

The real kicker came on day three, when Mom announced that Paul and I were to take Dad to his urology checkup. "It's just a follow-up. But you need to write down everything the doctor says because your father doesn't always pay attention lately." She didn't mention that he also might not know the current year as he filled out his intake form or that he wouldn't be able to tell the difference between a credit card and his insurance card at reception.

The urologist was surprised to see a co-ed crowd in the exam room — by this point, my brother and I had decided that all three of us should be there, and Dad seemed to have no objections, even changing into an exam gown in front of me.

"So," the doctor began, "have you decided whether to go ahead on the surgery?"

All three of us stared blankly.

"The biopsy. For the mass."

What mass?! What biopsy?! Dad was oblivious, and it seemed Mom had not understood the seriousness of the terms during their last visit.

The mystery mass would turn out to be kidney cancer that would kill my father in a few years — although the unsuccessful surgery to retrieve a biopsy, later that summer, proved so physically hard on him that we never found out for sure. Mom wisely refused to let the doctors put him through the stress of trying again, and Dad, when asked how he felt about it, merely shrugged. As happens with many people, his dementia fog grew denser after this surgery.

Meanwhile, Mom, the one with the broken bones that had launched this odyssey, wasn't doing so well herself. As she mended, I saw her lose her patience with Dad's endless repetition, his habit of saying "hello, hello, HELLO?" into the TV remote instead of the phone. Having also lost significant hearing, she'd shout at him in exasperation. More discreet, astonished glances between us siblings.

The few weeks of nursing her made it clear that my parents' days of living independently were numbered. One of us had to stay with them until Mom was back on her feet. Dad simply couldn't help her, and we were terrified of him driving. (Once a GM test driver, he must have sensed his ability was declining; he was docile about our jumping in the driver's seat, as my Mom had been doing.) But after she recovered, then what? How long could things stay in this new normal, or patched-up semblance of "normal"? What if something else were to happen?

The churning conversations began. I'm not sure any of us (myself included, despite knowing the most about Alzheimer's) fully grasped how wide the ripples of the downward spiral of dementia would be, how taxing it is on any caregiver, let alone an 80-year-old partially deaf wife in dubious shape herself. One sibling thought maybe we were overreacting. Another lobbied for wait-and-see. We entertained various eventual scenarios: Move in with me? A nice place near you? Assisted living?

"Oh, we can't move!" Mom said, quashing all of it. "It would kill your father!"

Flash forward less than a year. I'll never forget the sight of my smiling, widowed Dad sitting poolside in shorts and black socks on a hot North Carolina spring day, my brother's dachshund in his lap and a beer in his hand as he watched 10 of his 14 grandchildren splash about. Six months after the phone call announcing she'd broken her pelvis, my mom died of a recurrence of an earlier ureteral cancer that had fatally spread before it could be detected or treated. She got sick after Thanksgiving and was gone by Christmas.

That left my family, like so many families — like my Mom had initially had tried to do by herself — to figure out how to manage Dad's rapidly failing memory, odd behaviors, and childlike dependence. How to keep him busy but safe? How to help him feel calm and happy? How to cope with our own conflicting levels of denial, frustration, impatience, and grief?

It's about other relatives

We'd been through a version of this a few years earlier, with my beloved maternal grandmother. Gram had been like a third parent to the five of us kids, living just a few miles away throughout my childhood, a fixture at every family party or school event, large or small. She died of Alzheimer's at 99, just three years before Mom did, a very long goodbye that had ended in a nursing home.

My mom was her only child. I'm convinced the stress of caring for her mother without much help or much understanding of the disease hastened Mom's own death a few years later. This is common: Elderly caregivers have a much higher mortality rate than non-caregivers, research shows. They experience much higher depression rates, and their self-care is worse, a perfect storm for another unhappy ending. My mom was already run ragged by the time she'd begun covering for my dad, taking over more of the finances, driving, social planning, and other tasks. She first lived with the added burdens of being older and an only child, as a caregiver, then fate threw in the special stressor of watching her spouse's cognitive decline, an experience that's emotionally cruel in a way an adult child can't begin to imagine.

Meanwhile, at about this same time, my mother-in-law was having similar symptoms. She would die of Alzheimer's within months of my father. (My poor kids lost all three living grandparents, all they'd ever known, in one brief swoop.) In this family, too, siblings who were spread out across the country (and internationally) reacted in different ways, each according to his unique relationship with her. One wanted to dive in and solve all problems immediately and aggressively. Another moved more covertly, providing support in more subtle ways. There was massive disagreement about how she should be protected and what should happen to her home. Some still don't speak.

The stress of Alzheimer's care isn't just day-to-day. It snakes across state lines and family trees. Stigma is huge — in my mother-in-law's family, there was an unspoken reluctance to suggest this matriarch might have any hint of senility, no matter how outrageous the symptoms, and especially not to discuss it publicly.

Ironically, after my dad died, I divorced and remarried, and my new mother-in-law, too, had dementia. More worried and geographically widespread siblings, more medical issues, more care challenges, more divided chores and divided opinions. And another highly stressed central caregiver on whose shoulders the architecture of this complicated support system rests (in this case, my sister-in-law, whose parents lived in her home).

It's about you

Ultimately, I wrote this book because millions of family members touched by Alzheimer's are living through similar stories.

I continued working for Caring.com throughout my family sagas. So in short order, I experienced everything the website covers, not only coping with Alzheimer's and cancer care, but also navigating sensitive family relationships; arranging financial and legal paperwork; working with gerontologists, social workers, attorneys, and physicians; researching housing options; cleaning out a longtime home; relocating an elder; working with hospice; finding out how to write an obituary and a eulogy; the end of my parents' lives, from shoes dropping to unstopped grief.

And every time I researched and wrote an article or blog post, these experiences became layered with new wisdom. Each time I covered an academic meeting on aging or gerontology, gave a talk, or conducted an interview, I learned more. For six years, I worked with MDs, PhDs, MSWs, and an alphabet soup of other experts, as well as countless uncredentialed but often equally knowing hands-on caregivers.

Surviving Alzheimer's summarizes these insights and practical solutions in a way that's speedy and accessible. Because few of us has a lot of time and energy, even as we have a lot of questions, worry, and stress.

Alzheimer's and other dementias don't just strike a person's brain; they strike his or her whole support network. If you're like me and my family, you'll often feel at sea. *Surviving Alzheimer's* is the resource I'd have wanted to help me get safely to the other shore.

o o o

NOTES ABOUT THIS BOOK

If someone in your life has Alzheimer's, you probably want to know things like:

* What should I say the twentieth time I hear, "What time is it?"

* Is there a way to make bathing less stressful?

* Why does he or she wear the same clothes day after day (or rummage in drawers, make things up, or fly off the handle, or — you name the odd behavior — and what, exactly, can I do about it?

* How can I keep this person occupied today without losing my temper?

* How can I get him or her to accept my help?

* How can I get family to help *me*?

* Is it normal to be so stressed? Constantly? Is it ever okay to snap?

* And, oh yes, what's the difference between Alzheimer's and dementia, anyway?

You want answers and insights quickly, as these situations come up. Yet you probably have a full life. Time is precious. Although more information exists on Alzheimer's and other forms of dementia than families could find just a generation ago (thankfully!), accessing what you need when you need it can be a pain. It takes effort to sift through long pages of explanation or to scan scores of web pages and forum threads to pull out the "gems" that will actually make a difference in your everyday life.

Adding to the challenge of sorting out optimal dementia care is that there are so many different perspectives. Each expert has a particular vantage point, informed by his or her unique training and field (or personal) experiences. Neurologists, for example, explain what's doing on in the brain and what might alter it. Geriatricians offer medical guidance. Mental-health experts shed light on personality and relationship changes. Social workers, occupational therapists, gerontologists, nurses, safety experts, nursing-home workers, and researchers of all stripes have studied or developed the best approaches for different aspects of care and everyday life. Not least by far, experienced laypeople have their own hard-won personal caregiving stories that can instruct and inspire.

Surviving Alzheimer's sifts through the best of these diverse insights and "connects the dots" between their perspectives. From all those dots, I've drawn a road map to help you navigate terrain that's constantly winding you through surprising new vistas and stressful hairpin curves.

It's not just one story. It's the collective wisdom of many stories.

Theory is fascinating. Narratives are important. But nothing cuts stress like applying fast, clear, realistic, and practical advice that works.

A Word About Semantics

I've deliberately chosen to refer to *Alzheimer's* in this book's title because that's the word that most people know, and it's the number-one cause of dementia symptoms. Alzheimer's is named for the doctor, Alois Alzheimer, who first described this disorder in 1906. (Don't we all wish his name had been shorter and easier to spell?)

But much is unknown about the causes and process of Alzheimer's — researchers don't even agree that it's a single disease. We now do know that brain changes can start two or more decades before your friends first notice you're repeating comments and have trouble balancing your checkbook (*pre-clinical* or *pre-symptomatic Alzheimer's*). *Mild cognitive impairment (MCI)* refers to a stage of disease where changes in thinking skills are growing obvious but don't yet interfere with daily life, and not all cases advance to Alzheimer's. As problems progress, many cases called "Alzheimer's" are thought to be triggered in part by vascular problems (such as small strokes), or worsened by other health problems such as depression, diabetes, or alcoholism. And because there's still no reliable, easy, and widely available way to get a certain diagnosis for what we currently call Alzheimer's, many people never really know for sure.

We just know Mom forgets to turn off the stove. Bob crashed his car again. Granddad has begun talking to things that aren't there. Jane needs help choosing clothes, paying her bills, cooking, bathing, managing her pillbox. And we step in.

The advice in this book can apply to many different kinds of progressive dementias. (Although there are obviously some nuances specific to, say, Parkinson's dementia or dementia with Lewy bodies.)

Two more prickly words: *loved one*. Sometimes I use this phrase to describe the person with Alzheimer's. I'm aware that it's not always the case that the person being looked after is a beloved figure. Sometimes they're estranged spouses, or parents, stepparents, or in-laws with whom we have fractious histories. Unfortunately we don't have a crisp word for "person with dementia" or "the person in your care," since *caree* and the chilly *care-recipient* aren't widespread here in the U.S. So sometimes I go by the majority who do love their relative with the disease, and call that person *your loved one*.

Finally there's this word choice open to interpretation: *caregiver*. Most of us don't think of ourselves as caregivers. Though the word is how researchers and academics refer to family members who look after someone with dementia, research shows that laypeople tend to think the word refers to people who are paid to do the job, such as trained nurses or aides.

We tend to think of ourselves as daughters and wives, sons and husbands, friends and family, simply doing what needs doing.

I get that. But I use the word *caregiver* anyway — because it's apt and shortish and because, frankly, we don't have a better word. (*Carer* never took off outside the UK.)

Helping someone with Alzheimer's is one of the more stressful undertakings a human being can be thrust into. You can climb mountains in less time. You have more training for driving a car. You get more support when you download computer software. Unlike other tough jobs, there are no paid vacations or glowing reviews. Unlike the similar selfless routines of raising a baby, there's no diploma, wedding, or other happy marker of a job well done to look forward to.

I know this. And I'd like to make it a little easier for the MILLIONS of us struggling to stay afloat.

Please Send Your Feedback

Are there subjects missing that you wish had been included? Do you have a tip or tactic that has worked for you that you'd like to share, in the hopes it can help another family?

Please help others who are dealing with this disease by sending your ideas or comments to survivingalzheimers@gmail.com.

** *All of the names in the caregiver anecdotes in this book, other than my own (noted with the initials P.S.S.), have been changed, and some stories are composites.*

CONTENTS

"Devote what energies you can muster to being kinder, more understanding, more loving to those who are still on this earth and to whom you are responsible. And save some for yourself, because you will need it."

— *Jerala Winakur, MD, in Memory Lessons: A Doctor's Story*

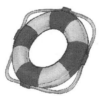

1 THE BIG PICTURE

Insights and inspiration from the Wizards of Alz

We all crave fast answers. That's why the bulk of this book contains practical, problem-specific, what-to-try-now tips and ideas. But first things first: When dealing with the sometimes maddening behaviors and situations that Alzheimer's brings, having the right perspective that helps guide you through the forest — and not just around each confounding tree — can dramatically cut your current and future stress.

That's why I've included this section of bigger-picture principles from the people I've come to think of as the Wizards of Alz, all of them amazing in their own way.

Here, meet some of the best thinkers in dementia care. Each carefully chosen expert has a perspective that's been shaped by his or her in-the-trenches experiences. Together, these views weave a strong foundation for your thinking and your actions as you navigate this new world you've entered.

o o o

Bob DeMarco: Step Into Alzheimer's World

While caring for his mother for 8 years, a son discovers a life-changing epiphany: Changing your attitude changes everything

When Dorothy De Marco died of Alzheimer's disease at age 96, hundreds of condolences poured in from around the world to her youngest son, Bob. "Dotty" wasn't an international bigwig. She was the muse, star, and object lesson of a blog that Bob had started to help himself understand his mother's condition after he moved to Delray Beach, Florida, to become her full-time caregiver. ("The world's biggest support group," he calls it.)

Alzheimer's Reading Room is now a leading voice for Alzheimer's caregivers, with thousands of followers. Bob, a former business executive and Wall Streeter, continues sharing the lessons he and others have learned as the site's editor. And if you think his site is rich with eye-opening tales, you should get him started talking, as I was lucky to do.

Most of the things caregivers experience at the start are negative reinforcement — you hear things like "Nobody survives" or you see how stigmatizing Alzheimer's can be. Everything seems to be going wrong, and you can't even control your own emotions.

I spent my first 18 months as a caregiver just trying to get a handle on what was happening. I'd stay up 'til 3 a.m. reading about the brain. I tried to adjust my life to take care of my mom. All my friends had always loved Dotty, but she had turned meaner than a junkyard Doberman pinscher. She'd resist me, argue with me, curse me.

Classic example: Dotty would open the freezer and stand there. She'd look through the food, open up packages, maybe re-wrap some (or not). Meanwhile the freezer would eventually start this incredibly annoying beeping, an alert to let you know you'd left the door open.

"Ma, what are you doing?" I'd yell from the next room.

"None of your damn business!" she'd holler back. We'd go back and forth awhile. Then I'd go in to close the door myself. She'd throw down the package she had in her hand and go curl up in a ball in her room. Things like this were happening every day.

Something has to change! That's what I found myself doodling on a notepad late one night. I circled the words and stared at them. I had no idea what it meant. But I felt the stress start to come out of my neck. I didn't even know I'd been that stressed. A few minutes later, I wrote:

And that something is me!" I circled those words, too, and then I connected the two phrases with a line. I still wasn't sure what it all meant, but I went to bed feeling unusually relaxed.

I'd made all our interactions about me — *me* being annoyed by the beeping, *me* getting mad when she wouldn't take a shower, *me* trying to tell her she just ate when she said, "I'm hungry." I thought I understood her confusion and was changing my life to deal with the effects of Alzheimer's. But it was all still about me. My mother was only going to change as the disease did. It dawned on me: What had to change was me — my reactions, my actions, my words, my emotions.

I had to enter Dotty's world — "Alzheimer's World," as I've come to call it.

If I'd had a travel guide to Alzheimer's World, these are some of the tips I wish had been in it:

- **Use the local transportation.** Before I interacted with my mother, I'd take a step to the left — literally take a step, as if I were walking into a new place. I did this to re-train my own brain to remember I had to enter my mother's world.

- **Speak the local language.** Eventually I realized I was drowning my mother with too many words. Sometimes, all I needed to do was smile. Or put my arm around her shoulder and my head on her head. Instead of a long explanation about what we were going to do (like go to the bathroom before lunch), I'd stick out my hand and say, "Let's go." And she'd come along willingly, even before asking, "Where are we going?" To which I'd just smile and say, "To have fun." Little did she know that I was the one who was going to have the most fun, after she took a pee without a fight about it!

- **Follow the local pace.** Everything is slower in Alzheimer's World. Have patience.

- **Stick to a routine.** Routine is key — structuring the day to replace bad patterns with good patterns. Build on what the person did before. My mom used to get up, read the paper over coffee, and run around on errands. So we'd do the same thing, only we'd go to McDonald's or sit outside, because I found that the bright light seemed to help her mood. We'd go to the gym, where the exercise made her smile and that brighter look on her face would last for an hour or two after.

- **Never forget you're in a new place.** So many people get hung up on thinking, "You're not the person I used to know." But that objectifies the person and distances you. It's saying, *you're a problem* instead of *we're in this new place together.*

So here's what I did about that annoying freezer beep: I stayed calm and took a step to the left. I tried to figure out why my mother might be rummaging around in there. I realized that her whole life, she'd open the freezer to look for something to cook later. But then she forgets what she's doing. It was comforting to see it this way. Or maybe she was hungry but couldn't discriminate between the fridge and the freezer; she'd open the freezer but nothing there was edible. Also, she either couldn't hear the beeping or, if she could, she didn't know what it meant, so it didn't bother her.

So I put a box of donuts, a treat she loves, in the back of the freezer. The next time she went in there, she eventually found it, took out two donuts that were frozen together, closed the freezer, and set the donuts on the counter. Later, she came back into the kitchen, saw them there, and ate them happily — without opening the freezer.

Instead of venting — calling my friends and telling them the same story over and over — or getting bent out of shape and angry, I became proactive. Instead of feeling burdened, I felt a kind of joy that Dotty was still using her brain to find something to eat.

Each episode like this brought the *positive* reinforcement I needed as a caregiver that my efforts were worthwhile — and I wanted to do more of it. The better I became at living with Dotty in Alzheimer's World, the more pleasant and cooperative she became. She still had her pain-in-the-butt days, but they began to bother me less. Something else surprising happened: I became more patient and easygoing in the Real World, too. Small stuff bothers me less. Let's face it, positive reinforcement motivates all of us.

o o o

Lisa P. Gwyther: Blame the Disease, Not the Person

Fear? Denial? Disagreement? This co-founder of the national Alzheimer's Association knows better than most that families must navigate an ever-changing "new normal"

What led Lisa Gwyther to create some of the first-ever dementia support groups, newsletters, and other educational resources for families about Alzheimer's? "They simply didn't exist when I started, and they were needed," says the director of the Duke Alzheimer's Family Support program and education director of Duke's Bryan Alzheimer's Disease Research Center. A social worker with four decades of experience in aging and Alzheimer's services, Gwyther is also an associate professor in the Duke University Medical Center Department of Psychiatry and Behavioral Sciences. She was one of 30 co-founders of the national Alzheimer's Association and is a past president of the Gerontological Society of America.

"Knowledge is power," is one of her many truisms — and the earlier you identify and understand memory loss and other symptoms, she believes, the better. I've often heard Gwyther, an inspiration to many in aging services, quoted at conferences. She and I "met cute": Out walking one morning, I recognized her — from her author photo on her book, The Alzheimer's Action Plan, *which she wrote with Duke's P. Murali Doraiswamy, MD, and Tina Adler — coming toward me. I'd interviewed her many times without realizing she was my neighbor!*

The disease affects everyone differently. If you've seen one family facing Alzheimer's —well, you've seen one family facing Alzheimer's. And the disease and families change over time, bringing new behaviors, symptoms, conflicts. Other unexpected things happen, meaning each "new normal" is only normal for so long.

People are surprised to hear that there's no one "right" answer or way to do things. There are too many variables involved. There are usually as many "right" ways to make a decision as there are families. You can only do what seems best at the time, in a situation often limited by circumstances beyond your control.

What trips up families most: They get mad at the person with Alzheimer's for the frustrating things he or she does or says and the personality changes they see. Or families get mad at each other for disagreeing about what to do, for not helping enough, for being too cheap or being too critical — you name it. But it's the disease they should be getting mad at. The disease is what's making their family member act in frustrating, intrusive ways and demanding so much of everyone involved.

Put up a reminder sign for yourself that says, BTD! ("Blame the disease!") It doesn't help to try to get the person with Alzheimer's to act differently or to extract promises about future behavior; he can't. You, not your relative, need to change.

There are no perfect families. All families disagree or have regrets sometimes. Most families disagree often. Alzheimer's can draw a family together or tear them apart.

Support groups offer something for almost everyone. Early stage support groups can be a relief and inspiration to people recently diagnosed (and their care partners). They're often social and supportive, as well as educational. Other groups are just for spouses, or for daughters-only, or men-only. People are sometimes skeptical or suspicious about groups at first, and it can be hard to get away to attend. But support groups provide a kind of compassion and camaraderie where everyone there "gets it," sometimes in ways family and friends just don't. Some groups meet online.

Support groups aren't for everyone. I've seen older men, for example, who respond better to the idea of attending an information session or seminar, like those hosted by hospitals or the local Alzheimer's Association. They're valuable, too. Some people aren't the type; they fear support groups will be like group therapy and force them to talk (which isn't true).

How to identify a good support group: Sit in on one, and listen for lots of "Ah!" and "You, too?"

Families talk about saving for a rainy day. Well, if you're dealing with Alzheimer's, it's pouring. Be sure you're seeking the appropriate level of care. Early in the disease, that can mean extra structured activities or in-home supports. Later, a common mistake is to think assisted living is the only answer, when the person with dementia may benefit from an adult day program or may need a secure dementia-care facility or skilled nursing care.

3 mantras to help you stay sane:

1. *The disease is bigger than me.* Define your limits, then call in reinforcements.

2. *Let's focus on what's left, not what's lost.* People with Alzheimer's have a lot to give.

3. *I did what seemed best at the time.* Don't waste limited energy second-guessing yourself.

o o o

Teepa Snow: Decoding the Secret Language of Dementia

The woman who might well be called "the Rosetta Stone of dementia-speak" offer insights on what it means when a loved one says, "That baby needs...," "I have to get home," and more

No one falls asleep at a lecture given by Teepa Snow, an occupational therapist and dementia-care consultant with more than 35 years of experience. She slips into character and invites the audience to role-play at her popular training and education workshops for professionals and family caregivers. Her goal: to drive home the lessons she's learned working with stroke, brain injury, and Alzheimer's patients, including her own grandparents. ("Although back then," she says, "they just said Grandpa was senile.")

The founder of the Dementia Care Academy [www.dementiacademy.com], Snow works with organizations across North America and teaches at Duke University's School of Medicine and the University of North Carolina - Chapel Hill School of Medicine. Not least, she has her own YouTube channel. Waiting for a plane one August afternoon that would take her to her 245th presentation of the year (she logs 300 travel days a year), I caught up with her on the subject of what the baffling words and actions of someone with dementia can mean.

Behavior "talks" to you. Instead of getting mad or frustrated because the person with dementia acts inconsistently or nonsensically, try seeing the behavior as a message. A behavior is like the tip of the iceberg — something to be curious about, to investigate and to explore, rather than to judge.

Say your frail dad starts to rise from his chair. "Don't!" you yell from across the room, "You'll fall!" He's telling you *this seat is not agreeing with me.* Or, *I need something.* Or, *I see something.* When you yell for him to stop, you're not helping; you're — without meaning to — making him feel bad (or sad or mad or scared) and he doesn't understand why. So he tries again. And again, you say,

"Don't!" He tries again, and you come over to gently push him back. He grits his teeth and says, "No, no, no, no, no!" — and finally, he hits you! Out of nowhere!

But it didn't come out of nowhere — he gave you lots of warning. Better to think, as your dad starts to get up, *Hmmm, what can he see from there that caught his eye? Is he thirsty? How long has he been there? Is his arthritis bothering him?* Think through what unmet needs he may have.

Communicating is like a treasure hunt. Too often, we want to get to the prize without having to go through the scavenger hunt of collecting clues to get there.

That's really hard for family members, especially, because we rely on old patterns to guide behaviors and communications. We also tend to have an agenda — we just want to fix the problem. We don't follow the other person's agenda, which is affected by the dementia. We rush to do things that need doing without understanding how it seems from his or her point of view.

We have to slow *way* down to communicate.

We're most comfortable getting messages across with words (and to a lesser extent, intonation). But with dementia, you lose vocabulary and comprehension. You hear fine, but by the middle stage of the disease you only understand every fourth word. Imagine I nod my head at you and say what sounds like (let's take away the consonants) *"Aeouoi ie?"* You might automatically nod your head back and say, "Okay," in a kind of social chit-chat way. And then you just sit there. But I was saying, "Are you coming with me?" And you didn't move! Your words and actions didn't match! As caregivers, we assume the message is getting through. We can't quite grasp that someone with dementia is no longer following those usual rules.

Always start with a positive physical approach: Connect first, then go to your "agenda." (Greet, then treat!) Don't charge in and say, "Mom! Your shirt is on backwards! What are you doing? Let's fix it. It's time to leave for lunch!" Better: Make friendly eye contact. If you open your hand near your face and then offer it to the person, it cues her to look there, at your eyes — she'll notice your hand and realize you want to come near and be with her in a friendly, familiar way.

When you get close, turn your body sideways, while keeping your face toward the person. (It's called a supportive stance, as opposed to a confrontation stance.) This way, she can see you're paying attention, but you're "boxing her in." Get to her eye level — sit or kneel (if she's sitting) or stand if she's standing. Say something like, "Hey Mom, it's Teepa." One thing at a time.

Then take a second to make a quick assessment: Is this a good moment or a bad one? Does she recognize me right now or seem aware of who I am? If not, she won't be very excited for me to start tugging her shirt off. It's about being respectful.

If she does seem aware, you can point to your shirt first, then hers, letting her eyes follow your gestures: "Oops, Mom, looks like you might have a coffee stain." Now gesture a "come on" signal, then say, "Let's go get a fresh one, and put this in the wash."

Try to avoid the words "Let ME HELP YOU"… it makes it sound like you think the person is incompetent.

If she seems distressed, sad, or upset, address that: Match your facial expression to hers and then say, "It looks like…" "It sounds like…" "You seem…." Be empathetic to make the connection before moving onto your agenda.

Five magic words: "Tell me more about that." People with dementia often have trouble coming up with the right word. They tend to get stuck at the noun. Imagine you wanted to use the word *coconut*. But you can't come up with it. You might describe it: "Like Almond Joy, like Mounds, the stuff in there."

People with dementia not only can't find the right word, they tend to lose nouns first. So they might say: "Round hairy ball brown stuff." I think, *Hmmm, something yucky?* I'm not going to hit on *coconut*.

Now imagine if I said, "Tell me more about that."

"Hairy in the brown ball!"

Oh, *in* the brown ball. I might say, "Show me that." Or, "Show me what that does." Or, "Show me how you use that."

You open your mouth. Ah! And I can ask more questions, like, "Do you eat it?"

Same thing with phrases you don't understand. A common one is *that baby*. "That baby needs help." It means, "I need help" or "I have an unmet physical need" or "I have an unmet emotional need." Another phrase used a lot, *I've got to get home or I want to go home,* means "Something's not right — I'm hungry, thirsty, lonely."

Repeat the comment and ask about it: "You've got to get home? Tell me more about that. Is there something you need to do there?"

"No, Mama's there."

"Tell me about that. Is there something you need from her?"

"I need to ask her what to do." Ah! This tells you she's not sure what to do or she's bored.

Tell me about it is a great decoder phrase: Tell me about that baby. Tell me about home.

Say she repeats, "I've got to go home, I've got to go home," over and over in an agitated way. You can tell from the tone and delivery that it indicates acute distress; she's not processing you or anything around her. In this instance, you could repeat what she's saying, following her rhythm: "You've got to go home? You've got to go home?" You telegraph that you get what she's saying, you get that she's upset. You connect.

Another break in the usual system of communication: People with dementia often get too close or touch too much. I come over and rub my hand on your shirt. You say, "Mom, why are you touching me?"

"Because you're pretty and I like you." I like it, so I touch it or I take it. I don't understand that it isn't mine. I lack that filter.

Or I see a child I like, so I start talking to him and patting his body. You say, "Mom, stop that!"

"But I'm just trying to be nice. He's cute."

"Mom, you can't touch him!" It's hard not to judge my behavior, but try not to sit in judgment. Understand that I'm trying to navigate the world around me and having a hard time doing so. When you point out my mistakes, I get flustered.

Caregivers tend to fall into the habit of seeing what's wrong and pointing out what's wrong, trying to be helpful when the person with dementia is making mistakes: *Uh oh! No, no, don't you remember? Remember I told you? Remember you agreed?* The word "remember" has no place in your conversation. They don't. They can't, so why point it out and cause friction?

Dementia isn't just a memory issue. If you just think "memory," you're denying the devastation the person is trying to live with. The person is suffering from brain failure, in two ways: 1) Structural failure, which means parts are broken and can't be fixed, and 2) Mechanical failure, where the wiring fritzes out — now it works, now it doesn't. That's why five minutes ago, it was, *I know who you are and why I need a walker.* But now it's "Who the hell are you and get out of my face with that walker!"

People with milder stages of dementia often have the hardest time because they still have awareness and memory present. They think, *I hate feeling stupid! I'm not a stupid person!* For some, the greatest distress is the thought that *nobody knows what I'm going through.*

They're doing the best they can with what they have left. Our challenge is to do the best we can to try to match up. Your flexibility is critical. Let go of how she was five minutes ago. You'll have more success — you'll be less stressed — if you can be in the moment and try not to judge. ("What a temper! She's fooling with me on purpose — she knows she needs her walker!") They're not doing things on purpose or to make you mad!

Trying to see it the way they're seeing it turns everything around.

o o o

Ken Robbins, MD: Be an Advocate, Not an Adversary

A geriatric psychiatrist explains how you can avoid those all-too-common damaging conflicts, arguments, and battles of wills

With his training in psychiatry, internal medicine, and public health, and a clinical practice specializing in geriatrics, Kenneth Robbins, MD, has been my go-to source for countless eldercare topics: stress, depression, burnout, resistance, anger, sexuality, incontinence, aging fears, grief, and more. My favorite (and one of the most popular with readers) was a series on how to talk to aging parents about difficult or sensitive topics. Whatever the subject, Robbins has the gift of being able to absolutely "get" (and explain) the needs of all the affected parties as he moves people from "stuck" to solution.

A clinical professor of psychiatry at the University of Wisconsin-Madison, and board-certified in psychiatry and internal medicine, Robbins speaks and writes frequently on psychiatry and the law, depression, anxiety, dementia, and suicide risk and prevention. You can read more of his guidance at Caring.com, where he's a senior medical editor, and at Health.com.

If you're dealing with dementia, you're probably going to run into arguments and conflict. You should just expect that, at times, your patience will be severely taxed.

There's a long list of reasons why: People with dementia often require constant attention, and that makes it difficult to get basic tasks accomplished — including sleep! What's more, the person with dementia is likely to be difficult to get along with at times. He's likely to have limited insight into his illness and therefore may resist necessary safety measures, for example. Most people with dementia also struggle with psychiatric difficulties, in addition to their cognitive limitations. Depression, anxiety, or psychosis are likely to make them very uncomfortable and irritable at times.

On top of all that, other family members or friends are likely

to have their own ideas of how the person with dementia should be cared for, even though they're not the hands-on caregiver. Hands-on caregivers often struggle with social isolation. The combination of the incredibly hard work, a lack of appreciation from the person with dementia and often even from family and friends — plus sleep deprivation — will leave even the best caregivers overwhelmed at times. It all makes it difficult to avoid conflicts.

If your relationship was already contentious, caregiving is all the more complex. When you start out resentful, it's harder to have empathy, easier to quibble. But even if you had a good relationship, there's more and more conflict as your loved one becomes more self-absorbed and says things he or she normally wouldn't. It happens to almost everyone.

A common, sad scenario: As someone changes, he says things he normally wouldn't, nasty things: "You never cared about me! You always think of yourself first!" And the caregiver is stunned. She says to herself, *I thought we had a good relationship. Maybe that wasn't real — he was just being polite all these years!*

Almost always, though, what's said in the moment does NOT reflect how the person with dementia has always thought. As the disease progresses, the person becomes more self-absorbed. As he loses more and more brain cells, he loses the capacity for empathy, much like a young child. If his needs aren't met in the moment, he lashes out with what he's feeling *in that moment*. It's not a broad commentary on you or your relationship. Too often, this wrong interpretation is what the caregiver remembers after the person dies.

All people with dementia become self-absorbed. You can't take what they say or do personally, because they no longer have the capacity to focus on anything beyond their own needs, much like a young child.

You never win an argument with someone who has

dementia. The reflexive way we all talk, when you know your point of view is more correct, is to try to reason. But you can't compete by the old rules because you're not on the old playing field. The other person is completely self absorbed and no longer capable of abstract thinking. No matter how reasoned your side is, it's extraordinarily rare that by explaining the reasons why something is unsafe or unwise, you'll convince your loved one.

Better: Talk about feelings. "You want to drive your car? Wow I can tell how much you miss being able to get around whenever you want. It must be hard. Let's talk about some ways you could get to the diner and the places you want to go." Acknowledge the feelings but avoid being an adversary. Gently redirect to safe choices.

The challenge is how to negotiate without becoming the enemy. If you're going to help, you need to be perceived as being helpful. Anytime you feel strongly that a behavior is unsanitary, unsafe, or otherwise problematic, it's wise to get a third party involved. This sidesteps nagging and arguments and instead gives you the ability to take the role of supporter, helping the person follow someone else's advice. That's easier with some big things, like driving or needing to move to assisted living, where the logical person to take the hit is the doctor. That frees you to empathize: "I sure wish you could stay in your home but the doctor says it's just not safe and I'm so sorry, but we have to follow what the doctor advises." Make clear that you're on your family member's side.

It's more of an ongoing struggle during the day with smaller things that are dangerous or not appropriate — the husband for whom chewing has become difficult but still wants steak, or the mother who wants to light candles, or the person who keeps feeding the dog over and over.

The obstacle caregivers face is that conflict can be continuous. It's your job to protect the person with dementia, so you have to say there are certain things he can't do. Try to arrange your life so you're not always the "no" person. Give "yes" choices you're comfortable with: "We don't have any steak today, but I can give you your favorite pasta."

A lot of people never get this new way of communicating because it's so unnatural! We spend our lives with someone having logical discussions together, reasoning things out. It's hard to stop! Your parent or spouse looks the same, but his or her brain isn't the same. You have to develop communication skills that are probably completely outside of your experience.

Endless conflict can slide into depression for a caregiver. Caregivers are twice as often depressed as non-caregivers.

Everyone needs to feel appreciated for all they do, but the person with dementia isn't capable of giving that kind of feedback. It's no longer a truly reciprocal relationship. Caregivers run ragged if they don't have other people to talk to for emotional support.

Here's something that happens more than you'd think: The caregiver brings the person with dementia to the doctor's office and tells him or her all the things that are going wrong. Under the circumstances, it seems correct for the caregiver to sound tired, irritable, and pessimistic — the doctor thinks *heck, I'd feel the same way in that position.* The doctor doesn't realize that the caregiver is in fact depressed, and that's why she's so negative and having such a hard time.

One of the cardinal symptoms of depression is anxiety and problems with sleep. You wind up impatient and just not able to be there for the person you're taking care of.

When you're depressed, you're not capable of being a functional caregiver. Learn the warning signs of depression (for a list, see the Resources section) and be persistent about telling your own doctor (as well as your loved one's) about your symptoms. Being a caregiver is one of the most challenging things a person can do — if you're depressed, that makes it nearly impossible.

o o o

Amy Goyer: This, Too, Takes a Village

Having the right support can extend your ability to keep going, AARP's expert on multigenerational issues knows — not least, from caring for her own live-in parents

Amy Goyer knows what it's like when your dad can still physically dress himself but can neither locate nor identify the underwear that you must hand to him. She knows what it's like to put off dental checkups for two years because you just don't have time, even though your teeth hurt (and wind up needing two new crowns). After years of long-distance caregiving — flying between her home in Washington, D.C., and Phoenix, where her parents live— Goyer relocated to Arizona in 2009 to be nearer them. In 2012, she began looking after them in their home. She's gone through everything from pneumonia scares and insurance battles to feeding-tube care and not always being recognized by her dad. (He now has moderate-stage Alzheimer's; her mom, who had heart disease, died at age 87, less than a month after our interview.)

And that's just Goyer's personal life. As AARP's longtime Family Expert, she's a spokesperson, popular speaker, and blogger who also consults with nonprofits and corporations. In typical working caregiver fashion, she wrote her second book, <u>Juggling Work and Caregiving</u> (AARP, 2013), by staying up until 4 and 5 a.m. for far too many nights. As she once told NPR's Jackie Lyden during a radio appearance, "I'm not just trying to keep my parents alive. I'm trying to have a good life with them and live my life at the same time."

You don't see yourself as a caregiver when you're starting out. *I'm just a daughter, helping Dad. I'm a spouse helping my husband, or my wife.* That's one of the biggest deterrents to getting support. "Caregiver support" sounds too official to apply to you. But if you're calling your parents long-distance to check on them or help with their finances, you're a caregiver. If you're doing what I'm doing, helping your parents manage every day, you're a caregiver.

There's a huge range of us. And we all need help!

Our normal support systems don't always adapt to our being a caregiver. I had friends who helped when I was sick or helped with yard work. But intensive caregiving? You can't truly understand, deep in your soul, what it's like until you've been there. The people around you don't *know*. They aren't vigilant about urging you to get out,. They don't know how to help. They get tired of listening to you vent or say, "I can't believe that just happened!" Caregiving truly separates out the dedicated friends and family members.

Isolation creeps up on you because you don't have time or you're too tired to do the things you used to.

The biggest deterrent to getting any help is that we're moving too fast! We're constantly bombarded with needs and issues and crises. There doesn't seem to be any time to stop and find support. Yet that's exactly why we need to see the value of it.

My doctor just warned me that I'm in adrenal fatigue from burning myself out — and I should know better! Like many caregivers, I thought my parents were so much more vulnerable than I was, so they needed all the help. Also there's a tendency to think nobody can care for your loved ones like you. This is true. It's also true that you *can't* do it every second — you have to take the risk to let someone else take part.

We tend to view help and support as selfish. It's not "doing something nice for yourself." Anything that helps you ultimately makes life better for the person receiving care. Dementia care is often a long, slow decline — and without lots of help, we wind up in a slow decline, too.

One of the most underutilized kinds of support is support for caregivers. When certain mundane tasks are done for me, like yard work, errands, cleaning closets, sorting mail, that frees me up to do more of the things I want to do for my parents. When I was looking for someone to check on my house when I go out of town, I discovered what's called a personal concierge, or sometimes a personal assistant. What a lifesaver!

The first reaction is always, "I can't afford that!" But for $12.50 an hour, one hour a week I know something that I'm stressing about will get done. For $12.50! And that lowers my tension and stress. (Rates vary by market, of course.)

Some other great sources of support that people aren't always tuned into:

- **Your local Area Agency on Aging.** It's the #1 place to call. See "Resources" They should be able to refer you to most of the agencies and resources in your community.

- **Home medical care.** Getting a loved one somewhere can be a huge ordeal. People don't realize that doctors who make house calls still exist. There are also mobile x-rays, mobile EKGs, ECGs, ultrasounds — all done at your home.

- **The Veterans Administration (VA).** My dad is a WW2 vet, but he wasn't tied in to the system. It's true that it took a year and arduous paperwork. But VA "Aid and Attendance" special pension benefits are designed for veterans and surviving spouses who need regular assistance for care. The VA also has a caregiver helpline (855-260-3274).

- **Respite care.** A colleague once cautioned me against using this term because people might not know what it means. I think it's more likely that most of us don't know how this *feels!* Respite care is when someone else temporarily looks after your loved one so you get a break. Adult day services are an overlooked resource for this; some specialize in dementia-care. You may also be able to find short-term stays in assisted living or nursing-care facilities. And some states have voucher programs where you can choose someone to provide respite for you, such as a neighbor or friend, and a grant covers that short-term care.

- **Supportive therapies.** I'd be remiss not to mention music therapy, because I started out as a music therapist. I've never come cross someone I couldn't connect with through music — and having your loved one occupied allows you to get a break. There are other specialists, too. For example, I'm also hiring the swim instructor from my parents' old senior community to work with my dad (and me!), as soon as I get the right pool rail installed to help him get in safely.

If you're working, be up front that you're a caregiver. Many people are afraid to share this. We're taught not to mix business with personal matters, not to bring home into the workplace. We fear we might not be seen as committed or reliable. But for the most part, it's better for your employer to understand why you're coming in late or taking time off — and you'll be better able to tap into resources and benefits your company may offer.

Start by talking to human resources. Ask what benefits and policies might affect you as a caregiver, including flexibility on hours, leave possibilities, and employee assistance programs, such as discounted legal assistance if you need to seek guardianship or a power of attorney. Ask how to talk to your supervisor about it.

Be very clear that, "I'm committed to my job," but without giving too much information, tell them the gist of your responsibilities. Don't overlook things at the workplace designed to support your health, like exercise facilities, gym discounts, or counseling services.

There's one more kind of support caregivers who've been there often credit for their survival, though it's not often talked about: spiritual support. So many caregivers describe this as a spiritual journey, in the sense of a life-lesson journey. They say that faith is the thing that gets them through always being on the edge of the abyss, feeling you'll never get it all done, never get the insurance paperwork handled, never get the damn pool rail finally installed right so Dad can swim.

Spirituality helps caregivers feel good about what they're doing. It can give you the faith that, even when things don't make sense, you can keep putting one foot in front of the other.

o o o

David Troxel: Give 'Em a Reason to Get Up in the Morning

Meaningful activities improve mood, cooperation, and even cognition — but planning things to do needn't be a burden on you, says this expert on Alzheimer's therapy

"Alzheimer's? What's that?" friends would ask David Troxel back in the mid-1980s, when he began working at the University of Kentucky Alzheimer's Disease Research Center (one of the first ten such centers funded by the National Institutes of Health). "There were no medications, few services, and little awareness," says the dementia-care consultant. But there happened to be, also in Lexington, one of the first day programs for people with Alzheimer's, founded by Virginia Bell. Frustrated families would bring in loved ones, warning, "Mom's so ornery!" or "Dad won't do anything!" Hours later, having done some art and exercise, maybe set a table or talked with others, they'd leave almost as if a different person. Troxel began to focus extensively on the idea of activity-as-therapy.

In 1996, he and Bell developed the "Best Friends model" for Alzheimer's care, which holds that what each person with dementia needs most is a steady friend who will provide loving care, accept their illness, and learn the "knack" of boosting quality of life. The duo also wrote the oft-quoted "Dementia Bill of Rights." Troxel, whose mother, Dorothy, died of Alzheimer's in 2009, is a past president of the California Central Coast Alzheimer's Association.

With Bell, he's a co-author of A Dignified Life: The Best Friends Approach to Alzheimer's Care, a Guide for Family Caregivers (HCI, revised 2012) and two activities guides: The Best Friends Book of Alzheimer's Activities, volumes 1 and 2 (Health Professions Press, 2004 and 2008). Though written mainly for long-term care professionals, you'll find the activity guides dizzyingly full of great ideas, including advice on tailoring them for different stages of dementia.

Why you don't want to flick on the TV and park your loved

one: It might seem easy, but ultimately, it's not helping you or your family member. People with early stage Alzheimer's have told us that they value creative activities as a tool for maintaining quality of life. All through the disease, interacting with others and doing absorbing things can improve mood, provide a sense of meaning and accomplishment — and enrich lives (theirs and yours alike).

Socialization is treatment for Alzheimer's disease. Boredom is the enemy. If nothing is going on, it often leads to the challenging behaviors that we see — agitation, aggression, crying, wandering.

It's stunning: It's been ten years since the newest FDA drug was approved. Even current medications for memory are modest in their impact. The good news, though, is that we've learned a lot about how to help people with Alzheimer's through activities and engagement.

I'm not talking about just being generally kind and loving. It's about building pleasure into the day. Use activities as a tactical strategy to foster cooperation and success as a care partner. This kind of approach can turn a "no" into a "yes."

Dignity is key. Keep things on an adult level. I'm not for crayons or baby dolls, which can feel demeaning and lead to frustration or anger (although everyone is different and some people are comforted by dolls). Think about your parent's or partner's life story and build rituals around that. Are their parts of their life story that evoke a smile or pleasant memory? My mother, a Canadian, loved a cup of Earl Grey tea with milk, and it would soothe her on a bad day. Maybe your mom loves to talk about her childhood on a wheat farm in Walla Walla, or your dad likes to revisit his famed hole-in-one and do a little putting with you.

People often ask me, "Do you think I should...?" And I usually say, try it! Want to take Dad to a ballgame? Sure. Have a plan B — bring a pal with you to help, be prepared to leave early. But don't fear failure. There's a bit of emphasis in the world of Alzheimer's care on "failure free" activities and sticking with what works, but I think people with dementia are like the rest of us — they like novelty. Always doing the same, safe activity can get stale and boring. It's good to be bold. (Using common sense, of course — maybe a 43-day road trip in a Winnebago isn't such a good idea!) You'll know soon enough if something isn't working. And you can regroup.

Start with categories of activities like these:

- **An ongoing project.** My all-time favorite came from a woman in New England whose mother loved ice cream. (Don't they all?!) One summer, she decided they'd visit every ice cream store in the area and create a scrapbook about it. They had their picture taken together in front of each shop, saved souvenirs like menus and napkins, and rated and reviewed each place. It was like their own Zagat guide. By the end of summer, they'd been to 23 ice cream shops and had a wonderful scrapbook to reminisce over.

- **Anything musical.** Lyrics can stay in the brain even after language skills are lost; music can be a real source of joy. My mother loved to listen to the 40s and 50s music channels on cable TV. I'd also rent old musicals on Netflix — if you turn on closed captioning, the song lyrics pop up. We'd have a sing-along. Later, when she lived in a care facility, I'd talk up taking her to a "concert" — we'd make ourselves nice to go hear, say, Luciano Pavarotti (even if it was just a CD playing in the music room).

- **Just being outside.** Take a walk, sit on the front porch, wheel your mom out in her wheelchair. You don't have to DO anything. Twenty minutes outside gives a day's worth of vitamin D.

- **Doing things for others.** When Santa Barbara neurologist Robert Harbaugh gives a diagnosis of

Alzheimer's, he also tells patients, "Now I want you to go to church / go to Macy's and spend your husband's money / volunteer somewhere." He knows that being social is key. Your mom might not want to do an art project, but she'd make something that was for her grandchildren. One woman and her mom baked dog biscuits for local animal shelters. Intergenerational activities work on multiple levels.

- **Simple chores.** People with dementia still need to feel productive — arranging flowers, sorting and organizing, folding clothes, hammering nails. When my mother was in assisted living, I'd keep rolls of wrapping paper, bows, and supplies in her room. I kept buying new things for her to help me wrap — for a friend, I'd tell her. She had so much fun, picking the paper, holding the ribbon while I tied the bow. Then a few months into it, she said, "Darling, I think you're spending too much money on your friends!"

- **Solicit advice.** I'd bring my mom half a dozen dress shirts and neckties, and ask for her help. She loved matching the shirts with the best neckties. It's empowering to feel you have a say in things.

- **Yes, exercise.** You already know the evidence shows it's so powerful; it may even be able to slow the progression of Alzheimer's disease. But one of the unsung benefits is that it provides small successes, a sense of accomplishment to take that short walk, or stretch with a therapy band, or do simple yoga. Bonus: Exercise builds strength and balance, reducing the risk of falls — and it's good for you, the caregiver, when you do it together.

Socialization and engagement shouldn't fall completely on your shoulders. Don't wait to tap into services near you. Look for an adult day center that has a dementia program. They're hard to find, but you're in luck if there's one near you. Or see if you can get someone with an upbeat personality to come into the house to talk and do simple projects with your relative, someone who's lively and laughs.

You don't have to structure every moment of the day. The idea is to improve your lives, not make it harder on you by being a one-person activity committee. Try to build in three or four anchor activities throughout the day, things that become part of your routine, such as a morning stretch followed by a favorite music show or nature video, time before lunch to play with or groom a pet, then afternoon tea or happy hour. When you think about your life or mine, we don't have every minute planned out — sometimes we're busy, sometimes we nap or just sit on the sofa.

Doing nothing is also doing something. People with dementia tend to want to be with you. "Activity" can sometimes mean just being next to you while you do your own thing — going driving, going to the grocery store (if Mom isn't an aggressive wanderer), or just holding hands with you while you sit and read.

Don't overlook simple pleasures. My mom loved nothing more than going for a drive and listening to old music — then we'd pull into a drive-through restaurant and order a hot dog followed by ice cream, so we didn't have to get out of the car and deal with waiting at a table and all that. Plus, it had all the winning elements many people with dementia seem to love — driving, music, and ice cream!

o o o

Anne Basting: Forget What's Lost, Enrich What's Left

Music, art, and telling stories can transform "sick" Alzheimer's patients into artists, says an arts educator

Early in her career, having won a yearlong fellowship to study acting and aging, Anne Basting, Ph.D., found herself in a Milwaukee nursing home. For seven weeks she struggled to spark residents' memories in creative ways — unsuccessful until she said the fateful words, "Forget about remembering. Let's make it up." The stories they spun together became a series of plays Basting staged — and the kernel of an idea she's since taken to care facilities nationwide.

The popular organization she founded and directs, TimeSlips, trains family caregivers and professionals in improvisational storytelling for people with memory loss. You can train yourself online at timeslips.org. She's also worked with the NPR StoryCorps Memory Loss Initiative and is the author of Forget Memory: Creating Better Lives for People With Dementia *(2009). She's currently working with multiple local organizations to use the arts to lift the lives of isolated homebound seniors.*

We have a tendency to see dementia in black and white, as if you are or you aren't. But after a person is diagnosed, he or she might well live 15 or more years. Clearly, that time is not all a meaningless void. People can have symptom-free days, hours, minutes, or seconds. Dementia is not about half full or half empty. It's not about black or white.

The experience of memory loss is gray. We need to get comfortable in the gray and keep our eyes and hearts open for moments of grace.

Memory is social. This doesn't mean visiting people more. It means reknitting them into the fabric of our lives. Too often I hear people say, "It's just too hard to be around him." "It's so hard to see her this way – I just can't go." And that is how — so simply, so gradually, so quietly — people with dementia lose their most valuable remaining thing — their circle of friends. Friendship changes with dementia for sure. But it can continue to yield gifts to both people.

The arts have an amazing power to reach people with dementia. When rational language begins to erode, symbolic emotional communication remains. That is what art is, symbolic emotional communication — sharing a vision of the world through gestures, words, sounds, images. Shared communication of any kind — through singing, dancing, visual art, poetry, or storytelling — can bring people suffering from loneliness and isolation into community.

Opportunities for creative expression allow the person with dementia to be not a patient who is sick but an artist who can grow.

Our first healing impulse is to work on memory. In the 1990s, when I was volunteering at a nursing home, I tried many memory-based techniques to get residents to engage in conversation. I got nowhere. Out of desperation, I switched to imagination — replacing the pressure to remember things with the freedom to imagine. What I learned: Lean less on memory and more on shared visions.

TimeSlips is a creative-storytelling method that grew out of that experience. It's something any family can do at home. You look at an image together and ask open-ended questions that encourage the person with dementia to imagine stories about it. Use all your senses to listen: What are her facial expressions? The gestures she uses? The sounds she makes? It also helps to echo — to play those expressions back to the person with dementia to be sure you're getting them right. (If she frowns, you frown. If she laughs, you laugh, too.) This simple act of intense, whole-body listening and confirming is an act of deep respect.

When a loved one has difficulty remembering a name, a face, a date, a story — try shifting to a shared journey into the imagination. "I wonder what the people in this picture were thinking about. What do you think?" Or, "I don't remember her dog's name, either, let's make one up." Just relieving the pressure to remember can open communication and connection.

You might think, 'Oh, my dignified father would never go for something like that...." But you'd be surprised. People with dementia start to forget their social role. They might not remember they're a spouse, or a parent. They need a social role through which they can express who they are, and the role of storyteller really supplies that.

o o o

Naomi Feil: Focus on Feelings

You can reach through confusion to make an emotional connection, even when dementia is advanced; this insight from a pioneering therapist is a gift that's changing eldercare

Naomi Feil, founder and director-in-chief of The Validation Institute, literally grew up among the severely disoriented oldest-old — in a home for the aged in Cleveland, Ohio, where both her parents were managers. Now in her 80s, Feil is a legend in dementia care. Her compassionate Validation Method (also known as the Feil Method) for interacting with older adults with Alzheimer's-type dementia has been widely used by professional and family caregivers worldwide since the 1960s. She's the author of <u>The Validation Breakthrough: Simple Techniques for Communicating With People With Alzheimer's and Other Dementias</u> (1993, rev. 2002 and 2012).

"People hear this is a disease that gets worse and worse and there's nothing you can do," she told me. "But hey, these are human beings with human needs." To see her in action (and bring tears to your eyes), search online for "Naomi Feil and Gladys Wilson," for a clip from the PBS documentary, "There Is a Bridge."

When people are very old and deteriorated, no one enters their world — they're often just sitting there. They will withdraw inward more and more, their desperate need for connection all inside. Here's a person who has worked his or her whole life, contributing their whole life, who needs that connection again to feel a sense of worth. They are longing for closeness.

Validation is a way of communicating with very old people who have an Alzheimer's-type dementia. It restores a feeling of dignity and self worth. It's a way of being with them, feeling what they feel. You pick up their emotions and reflect them back. People who are validated feel safe.

"What's the point?" some people think. Families are told so often by the medical community that Alzheimer's is a disease that

33

just gets worse and worse, that there's nothing you can do. It doesn't have to be that way! Even though people diagnosed with Alzheimer's memories and their emotions may seem gone, these are human beings, with human needs. They're not worthless.

Even with someone who appears to be in a vegetative state, you can break through.

My philosophy is that there is a humanity that binds us together. When people get very old and have advanced dementia, they go back to this basic humanity — and you can reach the person on an emotional level, because you're both human beings who share human experiences.

Family members often grow angry with their relative for behaving in ways they can't understand. Behaviors almost always have some underlying reason. The person has an unmet need — for example, to be useful and productive; to express feelings; to be listened to and respected; to resolve unfinished issues; or to restore a sense of equilibrium when eyesight, hearing, memory, or mobility fail.

People often use repetitive movements to express their needs, especially when they can't talk. Body movements replace speech. Women often sew. Men often use their fist as a hammer. Folding and refolding, such as a napkin, is also very common, and tends to represent a need to get safe and feel nurtured. Objects can mean different things for different people — for one man, I learned that touching a shoe symbolized sex with his wife; for another, a shoemaker, a shoe was about working.

Ask very specific questions about what the person is doing or saying: "Will it fit?" "Is it a miter joint or a butt joint?" That shows interest and encourages response. Use an ambiguous pronoun (like *it, they*) to keep it going. Specific questions with vague pronouns also are useful with someone who communicates with words you can't understand. For example, the person might say, "I wirld with the woomets." You may not understand what *woomets* are, but you can say, "Was it fun? Did they say anything?" When you ask in an interested, nonthreatening way, you get a response.

You may not learn the meaning of the action or what need is being expressed. That's okay. Sometimes you learn a lot. The main thing is that you're in communication in their world. That's a lot! The person is less isolated.

The best way to approach: First, take a moment to focus on your breathing — slow, deep — to release as much frustration and anger as possible before you interact. Use a clear, low, loving tone of voice. Harsh tones can make the person angry, and soft, high tones are difficult for many older adults to hear. Get very close and make eye contact. Eye contact shows affection and reduces anxiety.

Use words that get at facts, rather than emotions. Factual words are more nonthreatening and build trust. Ask: *Who? What? Where? When?* Maloriented people aren't interested in understanding why they behave the way they do — in fact, they retreat when confronted with their feelings. So rather than arguing, engage: "Who is stealing your jewelry, Mother?" "What does she take?" Draw out a conversation.

Another helpful approach is to rephrase the gist of what the person said with the same key words and same level of intensity: "You're upset about x. You want me to do y."

Events, emotions, colors, sounds, smells, tastes and images create emotions, which in turn trigger similar emotions experienced in the past. Old people react in present time in the same ways they did in the past.

To help ease anxiety or complaints, ask about the most extreme example of what's causing a concern: "What's the worst that could happen?" "Is that the worst [fill in the blank] that you ever saw?" Inviting deeper talk allows the person to express feelings more fully — and release them.

Match the person's motions and emotions — how they breathe, how they move their hands or legs — to further enter the person's emotional world and build emotional trust. One woman, a former legal secretary, made busy finger movements in the air. Instead of ignoring the behavior, her caregiver began air-typing, too. They made eye contact. "You can type how many words a minute?" asked the caregiver. "Ninety-two" the women said, with pride. They were the first words she had spoken since moving to the nursing home six months earlier. The validating caregiver established empathy.

When someone feels, *'I am wanted,* I *am needed,* I *am understood,'* there is a completeness. I know it gives me energy to connect with an old person this way, and it makes the other person feel the same.

Sometimes in someone with very little speech or no speech, you see a repetitive motion, moving the hands or rocking back and forth with the eyes closed. Maybe a tear is coming down. They, too, have a need that needs to be expressed. They've withdrawn from the world in order to nurture themselves. Approach from the front — from the side or behind can startle. Gently use touch if the person doesn't resist. Try different ways of touching; think about where a mother touches a child. For example, move your fingertips in a light, circular motion along the upper cheek— every cell remembers where your mother once touched it.

I often use music when speech is gone. Not any song; you have to know the songs the person knew. Try singing a song from childhood. For many people, religious music, even a simple old hymn like "Jesus Loves Me" or "Amazing Grace" can be powerful, because of the emotion and safety that's tied to it. Get close and use gentle touch, and sing, matching your voice to the rhythm and intensity of their motions. If they're flapping their hands energetically, be energetic. If they're breathing soft and slow, be soft and slow. The person may begin to respond to your rhythm and touch you. You may not get a response the first time, but you might the next, or the next — or this nonverbal person might even open his or her eyes for a moment and sing with you. You'd be surprised at the emotional connection you can create.

All this is communication. And the person is no longer alone.

o o o

Leslie Kernisan, MD: 5 Things I Wish Caregivers Knew

A geriatrician urges you to shift how you think about medical care after an Alzheimer's diagnosis; it can make a world of difference for your loved one and you

Knowing a doctor experienced in the care of older adults is valuable. Knowing a geriatric specialist like Leslie Kernisan, who also understands family caregivers' critical role as health-care partners, is priceless. She's one of only 7,500 geriatricians in the U.S. — about 10,000 fewer than needed to meet the current aging population's needs, and 25,000 fewer than the projected need by 2030. "As a society, we're depending more and more on caregivers to help us provide the care that older people need," she says.

Board-certified in both geriatrics and internal medicine, Kernisan makes house calls and offers geriatric consulting services to families in the San Francisco Bay Area in addition to caregiver education efforts and advising tech companies about aging. The former associate medical director of the Over 60 Clinic in Berkeley, California, she has a background in quality improvement, healthcare leadership, and public health, and helps teach geriatrics at the University of California, San Francisco. Not least, Kernisan (my collaborator on many caregiving articles at Caring.com, where she was a senior medical editor) writes two blogs — Geriatrics for Caregivers and GeriTech — and is at work on a book on how caregivers can use new approaches to better help elders with their health issues.

#1: I wish dementia caregivers knew... that what seem like "little things" can make people much worse. Untreated pain, constipation, too much novelty or stress, medication side effects — you don't think they're that big of a deal, but for an older adult, they can be huge. Often these "little things" make a person with dementia much more confused or difficult than he'd otherwise be. These seemingly minor problems can even wind up sending your loved one to the emergency room or hospital, which is a stressful and risky experience for someone with Alzheimer's. And that means another crisis you and the rest of your family will have to deal with.

- **Pay attention when** a new problem develops, especially if it's over hours or days. Whether it's something physical, behavioral, or with thinking skills, don't automatically assign every change to the dementia. Make sure something else isn't going on.

- **One of the biggest problems caregivers don't always act on:** Sudden worsening in mental abilities. This indicates delirium, which means there's likely something wrong, like an infection. Often a caregiver will mention to me at a scheduled exam, "She's been much more confused in the past week." We often discover a urinary tract infection or medication side effect, but it's not uncommon for us to find really serious medical problems underlying the new confusion. In one case, we discovered a large pocket of pus next to an elderly woman's lung, which explained her cognitive downturn. Don't wait a week. Don't wait until the next appointment you have. Call the doctor or advice-line that day, and be ready to bring her in *today*.

#2: I wish dementia caregivers knew... to have doctors re-evaluate the care plan for other chronic illnesses in light of a dementia diagnosis. Most older adults have more things going on than the dementia. Many of these chronic illnesses require self-care that can get hard when you have memory loss and cognitive changes.

- **Common examples:** People with insulin-requiring diabetes should be given a simplified insulin regimen. It can also be hard for people with dementia to properly take "as-needed" medication, such as for pain or for COPD; instead the plan needs to be simplified, or you need to recruit more help to keep track of how the person is doing and how often they need to take the medication.

- **It's not bad to simplify a care plan!** Most doctors can do this, but you have to ask for it because specialists, especially, are focused on the problem at hand for them. Ask, "Is there anything we can simplify to make the care regimen more doable?" Often, if this happens at all, it happens too late. That's a mistake.

#3: I wish dementia caregivers would ... get used to thinking about the real pros and cons for every aspect of care. I call these the benefits and the burdens. Many treatments and procedures are overly burdensome to people with dementia and may be less likely to help than people realize.

- **Here's a common scenario:** Someone with dementia is found to have a mass that's possibly cancer. The doctor wants to biopsy it and, if it's cancer, offer whatever treatments are possible. You'd want to ask: "How stressful will the evaluation and treatment (if necessary) be? What would happen if we just watched it? And what are the answers to these questions in light of this person's overall health?" If the person has been in and out of the hospital over the past couple of years due to congestive heart failure, for example, then a full-blown cancer work-up may not be the right thing to pursue.

- **For any major diagnostic procedure or treatment,** ask, "How will this help with my loved one's care overall? And what are the likely burdens?" This is especially true for same-day treatments that involve sedatives or anesthesia. Often these tests and procedures are quite stressful and even risky for people with dementia, but many doctors don't focus on this when they recommend the test. So you really want to be clear on how the test results might help you better manage the person's overall health.

- **Get the doctor to help you think about the big picture** of the person's health. Doctors won't always remember to do this. Specialists, especially, tend to focus on the specific problem you've brought to their attention and how to fix it. They each focus on their own tree, and that can be to your detriment, because you need help with the whole forest. You need to know which are the trees to pay attention to most.

#4: I wish dementia caregivers knew... it's really important

to have somebody knowledgeable about the person with Alzheimer's come to the medical visits. Too often, people with mild dementia come alone. Sometimes it's because they want to highlight their independence. Or it's just plain hard for the caregiver to come in.

- **The trouble is,** people with dementia often have difficulty providing doctors with enough information, or with details on a symptom or a problem. This means important health issues can be missed or not get properly addressed. Anybody, whether you have dementia or not, can have trouble remembering what the physician says. Everybody needs an advocate with them at doctor visits — but especially people with dementia.

- **What if the person doesn't want you to come?** Try to explain that you'd be helping them retain important information. But if they won't let you, or you can't be there, you have options. At minimum, you can write up your questions and concerns and send it to the doctor before the appointment. Some doctors have "Share the Visit" technology (sharethevisit.com) that allows caregivers to videoconference. Or you can ask the doctor to call during the visit or send back a summary in writing or via email. Another approach is to sit in on part of the visit but also to step out for a bit so that the person with dementia gets some private time with the doctor.

#5. I wish dementia caregivers would ... start the process of advance care planning with the doctor as soon as they get a diagnosis or know they're dealing with dementia. Good advance care planning should always start with conversation, reflection, and learning more about what to expect health-wise down the road. And of course, because we want the person with dementia to be as involved as possible, earlier is always better.

- **To learn what to expect regarding dementia,** consider watching videos online together of people with advanced dementia. They can be hard to watch, but they've been shown to change the preferences that people express in their health planning. Be sure to consider what other health problems, besides the dementia, might bring on a life-threatening crisis or cause real health declines.

- **The hard, overlooked reality:** People with dementia often have other serious illnesses that may bring the end before dementia does. For example, someone with advanced COPD who has a bad crisis and ends up on a breathing machine won't be able to tell you his preferences, even if his Alzheimer's is mild stage. So it's important to talk about how other major diagnoses are likely to evolve, while you can both discuss them. Someone who has dementia and who's on kidney dialysis eventually won't understand why he's being held down and poked, and probably won't do well.

- **Ask for help understanding the overall health picture.** Not all doctors are comfortable helping families with advance care planning. If yours isn't, try asking something like, "Before we do this paperwork, we'd like to review the overall medical picture and what conditions are most likely to affect him." Ask, "What might possibly happen in the next one to two years? What key medical decisions can I be expected to have to make in the next year or two?"

- **Revisit documents as the person's health evolves —** every time there's a major change in health that changes the person's abilities (like a stroke) or health trajectory (like a cancer diagnosis). Repeated hospitalizations can also signal a time to reassess the advance directive; people may decide to prioritize different things as a person becomes frailer or sicker.

So often I have families tell me "Oh, my mother did her advance directive 10 years ago." Well that was then! Now that she's in a different health situation, she – or her surrogate decision-maker – may have different ideas on what should be done in the event of a serious health crisis or if it seems some form of life support may be needed.

- **Of course no one likes to think about health crises** and how our loved ones might die. But in the long run, this can really reduce the stress on caregivers. One study showed that when families end up making decisions at the end of a loved one's life, the negative stress effects from factors like uncertainty and the logistics of decision making can last for months or years; advanced directives specifying treatment reduced caregiver stress.

Plus, it's important to try to honor a person's wishes and preferences at the end-of-life. Planning gives people a way to think about those wishes, share their thoughts with loved ones, and document them so that doctors later have guidance on what to do.

o o o

Barbara Kate Repa: To Protect Against Legal and Care Hassles, Act Now

This attorney and caregiver knows all too well that few families like to discuss the "what ifs" — even if dementia is the mother of all wake-up calls

For nearly 50 years, attorney Barbara Kate Repa has kept in touch with a dozen friends she grew up with in Wisconsin. This year, though, a third of them — including Repa — had to skip their annual reunion due to what they called "mom watch." Their mothers, nearing the end of life (Repa's is 92) needed hands-on daughter care even more than the daughters needed camaraderie and wine. "So many of us are in the same situation," she says, shuttling between Milwaukee and her San Francisco home.

Repa's career intertwines consumer legal education and eldercare concerns. She's an author of WillMaker, the bestselling software that allows laypeople to write their own wills, healthcare directives, powers of attorney, and final arrangements. A volunteer ombudsman (resident advocate) in memory care nursing homes, she's also a past president of the Bay Area Funeral Society and the California Board of Funeral Directors and Embalmers.

Despite her long expertise in senior legal issues, her own father, Frank Repa, had no will when he died in 2003. "Our Midwestern reserve got in the way. The dirty topic of who-got-what wasn't part of polite conversation," she recalls. In the long run, that thinking doesn't serve anyone. And in our family, the failure to face the issue of mortality head-on created a huge mess that took months to sort out. That could have been avoided if we'd just had a couple of conversations about it."

Why this stuff matters: I see some caregivers who have all their loved ones' legal and financial matters in order, with neat sets of matching file folders. More often, their heads are in the sand. What the ostriches don't realize, until it's too late, is that someone will have to take care of all sorts of legal and practical matters when their loved ones can't: ensuring appropriate medical care, inventorying and managing property, filing tax returns, selling assets — and after death, distributing property as the law or estate planning documents direct.

It's relatively easy to get things in order when your loved one is still mentally competent. But it can become a BIG headache if you wait. To put it in perspective, naming an agent in a power of attorney *now* to deal with financial issues takes a couple hours and often involves no cost. The alternative — waiting until your loved one isn't mentally competent to sign the forms and being forced to get an adult guardianship or conservatorship — can take time, cost thousands of dollars, and also sacrifice personal privacy as matters of mental competence are aired in court.

The two things most people need to think about are:

1. Protecting money and assets (with a financial power of attorney, to handle the person's money in his lifetime if he's unable, and a trust, will, or both that will take effect after death)

2. Ensuring appropriate medical care (through a HIPAA release, so you can view and discuss medical records; a medical power of attorney, to name someone to handle decisions when the person is incapacitated; and advance directives that express preferences, so you don't have 10 different family members arguing over what "Dad would have wanted")

Even through moderate-stage Alzheimer's, people can have the mental capacity to finalize these documents. (Not that you should wait this long, if you can help it.) The law generally only requires that a person understand what the document is and what it does at the time it's finalized. We all know that the thinking skills of people with dementia come and go; they have good days and bad, and they tend to do better in the morning than late in the day.

To help protect the legal validity of these documents, there a few precautions you can take. Put some thought into who you have as witnesses — don't just grab whoever's in the waiting room. If capacity might be questioned later, get witnesses who truly know the person with dementia, someone who can say, "Yes, I had lunch with Joe that day and he was lucid; we talked about the past and the future."

Making videos is also becoming popular. You can record the person saying something like, "I have strong feelings about my medical care, and so I'm making these decisions." Writing a letter, if the person is the letter-writing type and can still write cogently, is another way to preserve evidence you might need down the line to prove your loved one had the required mental capacity.

Even though I believe most people don't need a lawyer to help with many end-of-life documents, it's usually a good idea to get an expert involved if your loved one has been diagnosed with Alzheimer's, especially if you suspect any document might be challenged. No lawyer should finalize a document if she felt the person lacked legal capacity to make it, so a lawyer's testimony may be helpful evidence in case of a later challenge. It's best to find someone who specializes in eldercare or estate planning for an older person, because they'll understand the key issues, from Medicaid planning to practical ways to stave off possible family disputes.

Biggest source of confusion: How and when these documents take effect. People sometimes think that if they're named as an agent in a power of attorney document (for healthcare or for finances) they immediately become the person in charge. They think it means that they can ramrod through any decision. But that's not true. In most cases, the document takes effect when the person is no longer able to make decisions as certified by one or more medical experts. And it only lasts until the person's death. Check the document for specific wording about how and when it takes effect — or be sure to write one that takes effect immediately if that's what's required.

Biggest source of lasting family grudges: Disputes over money and assets. Like many other things, family fights tend to follow the money. Documents having anything to do with money and other property — wills, trusts, power of attorney for finances — are the ones most challenged, so make sure you get them right.

And there may be another reason to act to protect money and other assets: fraud. Unfortunately a lot of people prey on older adults with dementia. Lonely elders are vulnerable to a friendly voice on the phone or may fall into an old-fashioned politeness and not have the gumption to say no.

Often what's needed most is to get another set of eyes on an older person's finances just to be sure he or she is not falling for trumped-up home repair or insurance schemes that could deplete funds needed later for essential housing and care costs.

A financial power of attorney should be in place to make sure bills are paid, that forgotten bills don't turn into legal problems, and so on. The person named as the agent is often a family member but could be a trusted friend or even a trained outsider (like a professional fiduciary).

If you're the agent named in a power of attorney for finances, it's important to be transparent about how and where the money you're managing is spent. Make sure you fastidiously document expenditures, the inflows and outflows of money. It's easy to do with Quicken or other simple financial software. Or hire a bookkeeper if you're not good at it. You want to stave off any future challenges from anyone who might claim you were acting wrongfully.

You may be able to do a lot informally to deal with finances, too. The solution may be as easy as talking with the staff at the bank to get the information needed to monitor another person's accounts and expenses. There's supposed to be an iron curtain of privacy in finances. The reality is that if your situation is a known commodity, especially in a small town or where they know your mom and dad, bank staff may be willing to set up online access for you or send statements.

One of the great "shoulds" in life: We should all prepare a will. Yet more than 70 percent of people over 55 don't, an American Bar Association study showed. With dementia, it's a good idea to get an attorney's help to protect against future legal challenges. At home, you can start by asking the person whether he or she has ideas about specific people or organizations getting particular property.

The property covered doesn't necessarily have to be valuable; it might be something with mostly sentimental value that might get overlooked by others, such as vacation mementos collected over the years. It's a good idea to sketch out these things before you get to a lawyer's office, to save time and money.

You don't need a will or trust for everything to ensure there's a chain of ownership for property after death. A car and a bank account are the biggest assets many people own—and you can often simply name the next owner to take them by specifying a "transfer on death" or "pay on death" beneficiary. In most states, you can do this with a simple form at the Department of Motor Vehicles (DMV) for a car or at a bank for checking and savings accounts. On the owner's death, the property or money passes directly to the person designated rather than having to go through the time and expense of the probate process.

When monitoring your loved one's medical care, it's often enough to get a HIPAA release form to get access to his or her medical records. The patient is usually required to have some capacity to give access but doctors will often overlook this, especially if you're working with a geriatrician (specialist in the aged), who is more likely to bend the rules and have the attitude of "we're all in this together." A lot of medical records are now online — if you have your loved one's access info (including a password), that's a golden nugget.

Also, encourage your loved one to complete an advance directive or power of attorney for medical care to designate a person to supervise medical care and specify the care wanted if he or she becomes unable to express those wishes. The best help in resolving questions about such documents would usually come from medical personnel rather than an attorney, who doesn't know the person's symptoms and situation or the possible effects of various treatments. Doctors are supposed to follow all advance directives, but slip-ups happen. Sometimes family members don't know they exist, or medical personnel overlook them in a file.

As added insurance, there's another kind of medical directive, which is relatively new: the POLST (physician's orders for life sustaining treatments) or MOLST (medical orders for life sustaining treatments); the name given depends on the state. The benefit is that the doctor must also sign it, signifying that he or she will provide only the care the patient would want for both current and future medical treatment.

Another advantage: You can still set up a POLST or MOLST if your loved one is slipping; they don't usually require capacity, but allow another person to complete them on behalf of the patient.

Don't pay for documents directing medical care. The patient representative at your local hospital should be able to supply them, free of charge. You can also find the forms online by searching your state name, "statutes," and the type of document you need: power of attorney for medical care, advance directive, "MOLST" or "POLST."

o o o

Richard S. Isaacson, MD: Balancing Hope and Realism

Medicine and diet can't cure your love one, but it's important to know how they might help (both of you!), says this cutting-edge neurologist

Richard Isaacson eats likes he talks — that is, he follows his own advice about the increasingly promising benefits of diet and nutrition in slowing the onset and progression of Alzheimer's. At a dinner following his presentation at an AlzheimersDisease.com webinar for caregivers, he chooses the salmon and lots of veggies. He sticks to a single glass of red wine. He passes on dessert — although he's partial to dark chocolate and tells me he tries to get a similar dose of beneficial antioxidants with less sugar by stirring packets of dark cocoa powder into his morning coffee.

It's not just academic for Isaacson, who recently became the director of the first Alzheimer's prevention program at a major university, the Alzheimer's Prevention & Treatment Program at Weill Cornell Medical College / New York-Presbyterian Hospital. He has a family history of Alzheimer's. Also an associate professor of neurology at Cornell and director of its neurology residency training program, he's board-certified in psychiatry and neurology. His books include <u>Alzheimer's Treatment Alzheimer's Prevention: A Patient & Family Guide</u> (2012, AD Education Consultants) and <u>The Alzheimer's Diet: A Step-by-Step Nutritional Approach for Memory Loss Prevention & Treatment</u> (2013, AD Education Consultants).

Some families hear a certain drug can fix this, or they've read on the Internet that something like coconut oil can cure Alzheimer's, and they come to me to find out how much to take. At the opposite extreme, others come to me frozen with fear; they haven't been able to figure out about what they can or should be doing therapeutically after getting an Alzheimer's diagnosis. It can be hard for everyone to know what's realistic, what to try.

I always start by saying, "Let's take 10 steps back." Are you certain your loved one has Alzheimer's (and not another condition)? What stage? Does he or she also have other diseases? What are current lifestyle habits? I try to develop a broad management plan for that individual. It's not about one thing.

Unfortunately, Alzheimer's treatment isn't one-size-fits-all. It's not yet as straightforward as, say, treating high blood pressure. We can't just say, "Eat less salt." With Alzheimer's, there are more variables, there's more to explain — and the stress is higher for the caregiver, so there's a lot to talk about.

But the science is changing so fast. We're at the point where we know enough to say everyone can and should be using dietary strategies as part of a prevention or treatment plan for Alzheimer's or memory loss in general.

The big "but": How well an individual responds to treatments boils down to genetics. You can throw the kitchen sink at someone and see little effect. You might say, "My Grandpa did everything right, he worked in the fields, he never smoke or drank, and he still got sick." I understand that frustration. What we don't know is, if he had done everything wrong, might he have gotten sick five or 10 years sooner?

Different people will respond to therapies in different ways, depending on their genes. We know some people are clearly helped by diet and lifestyle changes. We just don't know yet who benefits most. There's also a lot of complexity in the dose, the duration, how you take it, when you take it — a lot of unknowns.

But the good news is that these are interventions with little downside. The risk is low, and the potential for benefit is moderate or high.

A lot of this is hot-off-the-presses data. Just five or so years ago, there wasn't much high-quality, scientific evidence that once you developed Alzheimer's you could change the progression by what you eat. But there's been an explosion in rigorous data, and now some of these findings can be put into clinical practice.

Case in point: A large long-term study published in the journal *Archives of Neurology* in 2012 showed that older adults who ate two servings of blueberries or strawberries a week (meaning, at least a half a cup twice per week) delayed cognitive decline by two years, probably due to the berries' high content of anthocyanidins, a powerful antioxidant. It's too soon to say how long you have to eat berries to see a benefit. But this data tells us that a diet high in flavonoids (tea, dark chocolate, citrus fruits, red wine) is good for the brain. And that's a simple change you can make.

No magic bullets: Try not to over-focus on berries or cocoa powder or some other isolated nutrient. It's likely a combination of factors within a healthy diet is what makes a difference in the brain. And the healthy diet seems to work in combination with other lifestyle effects, as well as your genes.

Some of the risk-reducing effects from dietary changes are as large or larger than you see with the current FDA-approved medications for Alzheimer's. But there are no guarantees. Just as no risk factor (not even old age or genetic predisposition) means an individual is necessarily going to develop AD, no protective or risk-reducing factor (not even a brain-healthy diet) can guarantee that someone *won't* develop Alzheimer's. It's about reducing risk and slowing progression.

Notice I talk about prevention and treatment together. Although there are some differences, many of the same interventions apply. So if you're the caregiver of someone with Alzheimer's, you're smart to adopt "treatments" yourself, because you're already at higher risk of developing the disease. And most of these practices can, coincidentally, lower the risk of other chronic diseases, like heart disease and diabetes.

My top five lifestyle strategies for preventing and treating Alzheimer's: This list might sound like you've heard it all before. But there's solid evidence that steps like these have the lowest risk and the highest potential benefits:

1. *A brain-healthy diet.* In a nutshell, this is the heart-healthy Mediterranean diet with a few tweaks: low-carb, antioxidant-rich, low-saturated fat, low-glycemic index, and high in omega-3 fatty acids (especially DHA and EPA). Basically that means: Eat less bread and sugar (which raise blood sugar quickly) and more carbs from fruits, vegetables, and whole grains. Have fewer saturated fats (like butter and cream) and more brain-protective fats (such as avocado, olive oil, or omega-3 fatty acids in fish). Eat more lean protein (like fish or chicken).

2. *Regular physical exercise.* Several recent studies have shown the positive benefits of physical activity (from regular exercise to household chores) in possibly reducing the risk of Alzheimer's and mental decline, even in people older than 80. Recent data has shown that regular exercise maintains heart function, and that alone relates to a larger brain volume.

More recently, scientists have discovered that exercise reduces the pathologic protein in the AD brain called amyloid (or beta-amyloid protein). Most physicians tend to believe that more is better. For example, walking just 20-30 minutes a day, a few times a week, can make a big difference, yet 30-45 minutes several times a week may help even more. As long as it's been approved by the treating physician, exercise is generally among the most important things a person can do to preserve memory.

3. *Cognitively-stimulating activity.* Music activities have been found to be especially brain-stimulating. People who have engaged in lifelong musical activities have been found to have added protection against cognitive decline and memory loss.

4. *Low to moderate alcohol consumption.* It's okay for you and your loved one with Alzheimer's to have a small glass of wine with dinner, as long as it doesn't seem to affect thinking skills or behavior. There's no evidence that drinking helps memory loss, though some research shows that one serving (women) or 1 to 2 (men) per day — especially red wine — may minimize the likelihood of developing AD.

5. *Social engagement*. Make time for supportive friends and family — even if it's just a shared cup of coffee with a neighbor or staying in your book club while caregiving. Think of it as buying time, not wasting time. Staying active and engaged in life, through adult-education classes, hobbies, and other social activities may synergize with a brain-healthy diet and exercise program to provide additional benefits.

Rome wasn't built in a day. Start by making the small changes that feel most do-able. Add a morning walk to your routine with your loved one. Have berries with your morning cereal. Find an activity that gets you both out and exposed to others.

Some people already diagnosed with AD would benefit from what I call the "early bird special" a few times a week — dining early and waiting at least 12 hours between dinner and breakfast. There's mostly animal evidence so far, but fasting can bring about a very mild state of ketosis, where brain/body metabolism produces substances called ketone bodies. Ketone bodies may have a protective effect on brain cells and also may improve memory in people with mild cognitive impairment or Alzheimer's. (People with diabetes should avoid this, as well as very low-carb diets, due to health risks.)

What about Alzheimer's drugs? Medications may help some people with AD more than others. Some doctors find them marginally effective, while others see greater success. Again, it's not an across-the-board thing. There are probably genetic influences we don't know yet. There are now drugs available that have been proven to work across all of the stages of Alzheimer's disease.

In addition, there's now strong scientific evidence to support use of these drugs over a few years. In my clinical practice, I've found that roughly 30-40 percent of patients stabilize at least for the short-term on these drugs, 30 percent improve, and 30 percent will continue to decline no matter what we try. In addition to improving activities of daily living, like participating in conversations and feeding oneself, I believe that these medications can take the edge off negative behaviors, like agitation and aggression — and that can help ease the burden of the disease on both the patient and his or her entire family

To boost the clinical benefit, I typically recommend folic acid supplementation to patients on cholinesterase inhibitors (Aricept, Exelon patch). Or you can eat more dark leafy greens and citrus to get this. The prescription-only medical food (Axona) is another practice that seems to be helpful in some patients with mild to moderate Alzheimer's with a certain genetic profile.

Unfortunately, it doesn't help that you can see ten different doctors and get eight different opinions. Some doctors say, "Well that study shows therapy x may only work in 40 percent of patients. In six out of ten it won't, what a waste!" But if four in ten benefit, that's higher than zero in ten.

You'll be hearing more about "nutrigenomics" (the relationship between food and one's genetic code) and "pharmacogenomics" (the relationship between drugs and one's genetic code). I foresee personalized dietary recommendations being given with increasing frequency as the science evolves: Imagine if your custom-tailored "prescription" could be filled at the grocery store as well as the pharmacy.

We all — patients, caregivers, and physicians alike — need to balance expectations with realism. Some people expect the disease to retreat; we know that's not realistic. The goal is to slow progression, to stabilize the disease for as long as possible (or to delay the onset of Alzheimer's disease). If you stabilize someone for six months or a year, or if you delay getting it yourself for a decade, that's a win!

o o o

Leeza Gibbons: Meanwhile, Please Don't Hurt Yourself!

This TV personality and Alzheimer's activist wants you to do one thing today: Move yourself up to the top of your To Do list

The oversize kitchen of her airy Beverly Hills home shrinks to cozy, coffee-klatsch familiarity as Leeza Gibbons leafs through a family photo album. She laughs about a leopard-print bikini that was a favorite of her beautiful mother — "a cross between Jackie Onassis, Cher, and June Cleaver" — who had insisted on packing it for her move to a care facility, "just in case." And Gibbons tears up as she recounts the day that "sassy, sexy," and beloved woman no longer recognized her. Hearing her authentic Alzheimer's tales, it's easy to forget that Gibbons is a media personality with a star on the Hollywood Walk of Fame, a face you first met in your own kitchen, on the TV screen when she was an "Entertainment Tonight" co-host and, later, host of her own talk show, "Leeza."

"Don't hide it. Make it count," Gloria Jean Dyson Gibbons had urged her journalist daughter upon learning that she had the same disease that had killed her own mother. So Leeza — whose current jobs include co-hosting the daily syndicated TV news show "America Now" and "My Generation" on PBS (for which she won an Emmy in 2013) — created the nonprofit Leeza Gibbons Memory Foundation in 2002. Its centerpiece: Leeza's Care Connection, community support and education centers for caregivers. In addition to hosting fundraisers such as the Dare2Care gala and caregiver webinars for AlzheimersDisease.com, she wrote <u>Take Your Own Oxygen First: Protecting Your Health and Happiness While Caring for a Loved One With Memory Loss</u> (LaChance, 2009) and <u>Take 2: Your Guide to Creating Happy Endings and New Beginnings</u> (Hay House, 2013).

TV host Larry King describes the Alzheimer's activist and caregiver advocate in terms anyone dealing with the disease would do well to emulate: "For Leeza, there is only one way to move, and that is forward."

Mom first began showing symptoms of the disease when she was in her late 50s. One day she confessed to my Dad that she had paid the same household bill three times. After that, we all started noticing things about her behavior that just "weren't Mom."

She started using profanity — after never having cursed a day in her life. She repeated herself. She made paranoid, outlandish accusations to Dad, saying that he had never loved her and was going to kill her. (He adored her.)

We thought maybe it was alcoholism — though she was just a social drinker. We were in a state of denial. Maybe it was a combination of Dad covering up for her behavior and our not really understanding what was wrong. I guess none of us wanted to believe that our wonderful mother might have such a terrible illness.

I wish I'd known what a marathon this is. Battling Alzheimer's disease is an endurance race, the likes of which I could never have imagined. My mom was diagnosed young, at 63. She died young, at 72. In between, as Nancy Reagan says, it really was the "longest goodbye."

This thief of life, thief of memories, isn't content to take just the diagnosed individual — it wants the whole family. It can suck you into a deep, dark hole unless you take steps to bolster yourself physically, spiritually, and emotionally. I was distressed to learn that stress-related disorders can take 10 years off a caregiver's life, and that caregivers often experience so many stress-related challenges that they get sick and die before the one they're caring for.

Compassion fatigue is a very real syndrome, and it can take down the best. At Leeza's Care Connection, we say you should "take your oxygen first," meaning: Nourish yourself before you take care of anyone else. Keep your body strong; give your soul some strength, too. Take a break. Forgive yourself, forgive others; forgive again. Do those things first.

The ultimate loving act, the ultimate selfless act is to first love yourself enough to care for yourself — think of it as an investment that will allow you to love and support the person who's sick. When I felt my reserves were depleting, I'd remind myself to stop achieving and start receiving.

The caregiving challenge became hardest for my father, as my mother's disease progressed. I worried about Dad when Mom could no longer express her appreciation or her love but instead lashed out with anger at almost everything. I worried about Dad when Mom would turn around in the kitchen with a spatula in her hand and start swinging at him. I worried about Dad every night when he would go to his room and close the door, knowing we were losing him along with my mother. They were married for 55 years, but ten of them were stolen by Alzheimer's disease.

If you tore a page from my diary from this period, it would be shocking. Every day I felt frustrated and angry by some new change or behavior. I'd lose my temper. I'd make mistakes. I'd feel overwhelmed. I was snapping at my kids, getting distracted by everything. I began to wonder what on earth had happened to the old me and if she was ever going to return.

Nobody is a natural-born Florence Nightingale or Mother Teresa all the time. I know I wasn't. I'd look at other people and think they had so much wisdom and patience, and then there was me — I was *so* not those things! But I learned that no one takes their first step on this path with all the answers. Heck, I didn't even know most of the questions. Here's the thing: Being a caregiver allows you to either come face-to-face with the truth that we are all perfectly imperfect, facing vulnerabilities that are better handled with support — OR you can use your situation as a reason to prove that life isn't fair, that no one understands, and that you have to do everything yourself.

Guilt can become a constant companion. I've never met a caregiver who didn't feel some of it. So recognize it and let it go. When I was with my mom, I felt guilty that I wasn't going to see her enough. When I was away from her, I felt guilty for not being there. If I was out laughing and enjoying my life, I'd feel guilty because I knew Mom couldn't enjoy her life. If my sister was spending more time with Mom, I'd feel guilty. I'd even feel guilty because I was healthy and she was sick! It helped me to repeat to myself a little mantra I made up: "I love my mother; I'm doing the best I can."

More of my favorite self-care advice:

- **When someone asks if you need anything, get comfortable saying yes** — and provide a list for them to choose from. Don't be afraid to let people know what's helpful to you.

- **Break your responsibilities into bite-sized chunks.** Make lists: What do I have to do just today, just this week. Promise me you'll put yourself high on those lists, each day, by doing small things that cover the basics of being good to yourself physically and emotionally.

- **Don't ignore sleep. (Remember sleep?!)** Not getting enough of it undermines everything. Try a bedtime ritual like tea or a short walk to signal it's time to let it go. If your loved one keeps you up more than three times a week, keep a notebook of what's going on so you can look for patterns and bring this information to the doctor.

- **Get empowered by those who have been through it before.** Maybe your "team" won't be made up of the usual suspects; look for people who have patience, who allow you to be completely honest, who have been there, too.

- **Become an optimist.** I know it sounds counterintuitive, because you hear so much that may seem hopeless. But the lens through which you create your world affects everything — those glass-is-half-full people really have an advantage. Know that you can do it. Thousands of people have.

- **This one's from my Dad. He should know:** "Worrying about what will decline next or wishing you could recapture something from the past will only prevent you from being in the present moment. Even as flawed and difficult as it may be, that's where life is."

o o o

"Realize it takes two to tango — or tangle"

— Teepa Snow, occupational therapist

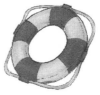

2 EVERYDAY PROBLEMS

Why they happen, practical solutions

My friend Rachel called, obviously upset. She and her family had just taken their mom, Ann, out to brunch — and for most of the meal everyone was happy and relaxed, she said.

On her way to the restroom, though, Rachel's mom stopped at the next table to coo over a baby with bright copper ringlets. "Oh, I just love a baby with red hair! I was born a redhead," Rachel overheard her say, patting the baby's head. "But when she hits the temper tantrum stage, look out!' Everyone laughed."

On the way back from the restroom, Ann again stopped at the baby's table — and repeated her earlier comment, word-for-word. This time the young couple just smiled politely. Rachel spirited her mom back to her seat.

"And then a few minutes later," Rachel told me, now getting teary, "Mom got out of her seat to go pat that baby's hair for a third time and told them the exact same story."

This time, the baby's parents seemed kind of freaked out by this strange woman who kept touching their baby. They pulled the baby away. Ann's family was stricken, too. They'd been noticing signs of forgetfulness but had never seen her do anything like that before.

"I apologized and hustled Mom out of the restaurant," Rachel said. "We were just finishing our coffee, but I was too embarrassed to stay. She was so mad, and kept saying, 'Why are you being so rude to this young couple? I don't want to leave!'

"I didn't know what to do."

Maybe you've already had an experience like that, or maybe it's farther down the road for you. Dementia places families in so many strange new situations of all kinds — it's natural not to know how to react at first. Often the best response goes against your normal instincts. It's easy to lose your temper, for example, but getting angry only makes the person with Alzheimer's feel (and often act) worse.

This section highlights many of these problems, from the mildly frustrating (like repeating stories and acting odd in public) to the downright scary (like aggression or wandering away). For each, I offer what I call the "Why-This, Try-This" approach to problem-solving. "Why" is an often overlooked, yet relevant and, to me, incredibly inspiring word in dementia care. Understanding some of the reasons behind what seems like an "unreasonable" behavior can help you extend your patience as it lifts your confidence. And valuably, pausing to think about the WHY can give you much-need clues on what you can TRY to prevent or change what's happening.

These problems and behaviors unfold differently for everyone. The following Why- This, Try-This suggestions aren't so much absolute solutions as tried-and-true ideas, rooted in an understanding of the disease and behavioral triggers, that just might help make a difference in your situation.

o o o

PERSONALITY CHANGES

How Dementia Can Alter Personality

Even before memory problems become exasperatingly obvious, family members often notice that a loved one seems "different" or "not himself." From early in the disease process, brain changes can result in noticeable alterations in personality (which experts define as the sum of temperament, disposition, character, typical thought or activity patterns, and other traits that make an individual distinct).

Often families see these changes but don't connect them to dementia. It's easy to believe a different problem is going on. A spouse might complain that a mate is growing rude or grumpy, for example — and the pair may bicker or grow apart. Adult children wonder if Mom's spaciness means she's drinking too much, or they take Dad's lack of interest in everything as a sign that he's bored by retirement. Actions that are the direct result of brain impairment are instead perceived as being done "on purpose."

None of these misperceptions are anyone's fault. Denial, confusion, and even sheer surprise about cognitive impairment are widespread and deep.

There's no single pattern of personality change in Alzheimer's. These four general patterns of change are most common:

1. Happy, in-the-moment

2. Depressed and/or anxious

3. Apathetic (unmotivated, uninterested, unemotional)

4. Paranoid, frightened, and angry

Consider them as four general "buckets" of demeanors and behaviors. But there can be individual differences, and there can be some overlap between them.

The personality you see may be similar to the person's pre-dementia personality. In many instances, though, it feels like your loved one has had a personality transplant. Also, someone might start out one way and shift later. For example, depression and anxiety in the early stages of the disease may mellow into a disposition that's more content as awareness wanes.

It's useful to know that such patterns exist, because they can help you understand why your loved one is saying and doing the things that are so out of character. You can better prepare for what might be coming and find ways to manage things and make life more comfortable for your loved one and you. And you'll be less likely to blame yourself for behaviors and incidents that don't really have anything to do with you personally.

Below you'll find detailed information about each of the four common patterns. Following these descriptions, the rest of the section offers advice on the specific ways these personalities manifest themselves.

o o o

Dementia Personality Pattern: Happy, In-the-Moment

My mother-in-law, Louie, was a classic Southern "steel magnolia." With her honeyed mid-Georgia accent, charm, and perfect manners, you might mistake her for just another pushover, a pretty flower. Once you got to know her, though, you saw that beneath this belle-veneer was a prickly lady of strong opinions and high expectations who wasn't afraid to pick a fight or hold a grudge. (I loved her!)

A funny thing happened as her dementia progressed, however. She became milder, mellower, easier-going. She seemed to let go of her need to control. When my son showed up with shaggy hair, there were no lectures about haircuts, just sweet-talk about how cute he was. When my daughters shifted from smocked dresses to short skirts, she applauded their taste instead of frowning. Once Waspily standoffish, she grew more huggy. More shockingly, she let other people clean up or do the dishes! She seemed happy just to...be.

That surprised me because Alzheimer's had turned my grandmother, who'd always had a softer, jollier personality than Louie, into a crotchety, sad shell by the end. My father, on the other hand, had lived his whole life happy-go-lucky, and stayed that way throughout his dementia slide. — P.S.S.

What it looks like:

Sometimes called "pleasant dementia," this is perhaps the least problematic of problems personality changes can bring. People in this category tend to behave in ways that are docile and agreeable. They generally go along with suggestions. They're polite, expressing gratitude and thanks. They don't seem to fret about the past or what's next; instead they take each moment as it comes. This ability to live in the moment seems to keep their mood relatively light, especially if they feel secure, loved, and well cared for.

"The burden of having to anticipate the future and prepare for it, and the burden of remembering things they don't like about the past, has been removed because of their cognitive impairments," says geriatric psychiatrist Ken Robbins. "They're now able to live in the moment and enjoy it." Sometimes the person seems happier than she's ever been.

TRY this:

- Do all you can to help the person have a stable existence rich with security and routine. This kind of care seems to help foster a calm, happy persona. (If your loved one doesn't show this pattern, don't blame yourself. Although quality of care influences behavior patterns and persona, it's not the whole story. Brain changes often trump good intentions and good care.)

- Be generous with physical affection. Hugs and hand-holding speak louder than words in creating security.

- Continue to find stimulating activities and social outlets for your loved one. Because this type tends to be so agreeable and uncomplaining, it's easier to forget that they still have a need for stimulation and guidance.

To help you cope:

- Allow yourself to experience the confusing stew of emotions these changes can bring. I remember feeling a mix of relief (an easy personality is, well, easier than a querulous one), guilt (for feeling relief), sadness (because I missed the sharpness and the person I'd known), and a kind of bittersweet gratitude (because my mother-in-law was no longer aware of her deficits and seemed to be enjoying life as it was).

- Take solace in the comparison that some researchers have drawn between pleasant dementia and that state of mind learned through meditation and mindfulness. Its emphasis is on acceptance, letting go, being fully present. It's ironic that a loved one's reduced cognition should help show us the way: *What a beautiful sunset...I'm not mad at you anymore...no complaints here...why thank you....taking the scenic route...Who, me worry?*

o o o

Dementia Personality Pattern: Depressed and/or Anxious

Ron felt he was slipping up. At first he blamed newfangled office procedures, or maybe it was just a matter of getting older. It was becoming harder to concentrate at work. He missed a few deadlines. When he found it hard to track his business expenses, he quit turning in expense reports at all. ("It's not that much money," he told himself. But he never told his wife, Tracy.) Once he got confused in the Atlanta airport; for the life of him, he couldn't figure out where he was supposed to go. Eventually he tried to board the wrong flight. He missed the right one and might never have gotten home at all if he hadn't run into Bob from the team. That was embarrassing, but it sure was a lifesaver. After that, Ron avoided travel assignments.

He felt best in the evening, with a glass of bourbon in his hand and a sports show on TV. Then he could relax. When Tracy tried to talk to him about her concerns — she said he wasn't paying attention to her, harping about that fender bender again, nagging him to see the doctor about working too hard — he tuned her out.

Tracy, for her part, noticed Ron drinking more regularly. He seemed to be retreating inward, turning down social engagements and not going on as many business trips. She worried about how his job was going. She worried about his driving — two minor accidents and two tickets in the last six months. But when she tried to get him to talk about anything, he cut her off. "Do you think I'm a moron?" he'd snap. "Leave me alone!"

Then he'd start muttering about crazy drivers and inept colleagues in a fretful tone, and take another deep sip of bourbon.

What it looks like:

Depression and anxiety are especially common in the earlier-stages of Alzheimer's disease, when the person still has enough insight intact to be aware that he's having increasing difficulty with his thinking skills. They may intensify as the disease progresses.

Imagine knowing something's wrong that you can't necessarily put your finger on, and worse, can't control. Nagging fears and unease begin to take over and leave you upset or down.

Feeling anxious about life (in general, or about specific incidents) causes the person to act irritable and fretful. He may express worry, fear, or dread, and have a hard time concentrating. Sleep may be affected. Physically, he may complain of headaches or stomachaches, and might tremble, sweat, or seem jumpy.

Associated behaviors include agitation, pacing, shadowing (closely following) a family member, hoarding, and avoiding be left alone.

Anxiety can slide into depression, or one can exist separate from the other, although their origins are similar. Depression can intensify memory problems.

Signs of dementia are similar to those in people without dementia: Changes in sleep (too much or too little), changes in appetite (eating too much or too little), loss of pleasure in things, a sense of hopelessness or worthlessness, sadness, agitation, and thoughts of death or suicide. (People with dementia who are depressed both tend to talk about suicide and follow through less often than the rest of the population.)

Up to one in five people with dementia have an anxiety disorder, and almost three in four are thought to have anxiety symptoms. As many as half of people diagnosed with Alzheimer's show at least some signs of depression, and the depression can persist throughout the disease. (Depression is also a risk factor for developing Alzheimer's; people who struggled with untreated depression before dementia may continue to have it as a co-existing disease.)

TRY this:

- Report symptoms to the person's doctor. It's important to rule out other causes (such as a drug reaction or infection). Antidepressant medications are used to treat both anxiety and depression. Sometimes anti-anxiety medications are used on a short-term basis, but they tend to have side effects, including worsening memory and a greater risk of falls. That's why behavioral solutions tend to be best with anxiety.

- Make sure he engages with others, since social isolation is known to feed anxiety and depression. Involvement in an early stage support group (for people with dementia) can provide both a social outlet and a safe place to talk about the stresses of adjusting to cognitive changes. Adult day centers are similarly helpful. Talk therapy can also help and at least some visits are covered by most insurance plans.

- Be sure he gets exercise every day, both to help mood and any sleep problems he may be having.

- Minimize traumatic changes. Moving, a hospitalization, or the loss of a consistent care partner can all intensify anxiety or depression. As much as is plausible, it helps to keep to a supportive, consistent routine.

- Step back to see if you notice patterns or triggers when behaviors worsen. Each person tends to have his own triggers: bathing, talking about money, or being overwhelmed by too many people or frustrated by not being able to do a former task to one's former standards, for example. When you discover a trigger, try to take extra steps to remove it (no money talk, no big parties) or make it easier and less stressful to manage (introduce a different hobby, simplify bathing).

- Help your loved one feel busy and productive. A sense of accomplishment, meaning, and purpose are critical to someone in the throes of anxiety or depression because of perceived losses (of ability, thinking skills, and auto freedom, among others. One French study exposed people with anxiety, depression, and dementia to cooking, baking, and music. After four weeks, their symptoms decreased. If your loved one can no longer work, look for volunteer outlets where he can channel his energy safely, rather than switching to doing nothing. Don't take over all the chores; let your loved one participate.

- Set up a win-win environment, where challenges and frustrations are minimized. Make it easy for him to find food and clothing and navigate through the day. Help in an unobtrusive way.

To help you cope:

- Realize that you'll need to play a fairly active role in managing this personality change, so gear up with all the help and resources you can. Part of the challenge in this situation is that coping with feelings of anxiety or depression is hard for anyone (you may even be struggling with this yourself). But when you're cognitively impaired, you're virtually unable to drag yourself to a therapist, connect with a doctor or an old friend you can confide in, and so on. Intervening and reassuring is an added burden on family caregivers, but your efforts can pay off in fewer disruptive behaviors down the road.

- Expect mood swings or angry outbursts — and when they happen, don't take them personally. Remind yourself of Duke's Alzheimer's Research Center education director Lisa Gwyther's adage: "It's the disease, not the person."

o o o

Dementia Personality Pattern: Apathetic (Unmotivated, Uninterested, Unemotional)

Gloria's frustrations with her husband's personality reached their peak the day their daughter brought the children over for Jack's birthday. Twins Ava and Aiden, 8, had made their "Gramps" a paper crown and helped to decorate his cake. They'd each picked out presents for him and couldn't wait to divulge their contents soon after they'd burst into the house.

"Whoa!" she said with a smile, bending down to hug each of them as they gibbered with excitement. Jack, who'd once loved spending hours teaching the kids how to tie nautical ropes or take care of his sailboat, never rose from his chair. He seemed to watch them all as if they were far, far away.

"Gramps! Gramps! Guess what we got you?!" Aiden shouted as he clambered onto his lap. "Hey! Gramps? Where are you going?"

To everyone's surprise, Jack had brushed off the hugs and hellos — and the grandchild on his lap. He stiffly rose from his recliner. Waving his hand back at the group, he shuffled out of the room. "I don't want any birthday."

Even the children just stared in astonishment.

What it looks like:

Also described as stunted emotions or a loss of motivation and interest in the world, this change tends to be readily recognized by family members early in the disease — though at first it might be mistaken for stubbornness, rudeness, laziness, or depression. Your loved one may be passive and lethargic, withdrawing from former interests or showing little initiative in making plans or following through. Caregivers often describe "something missing" from their loved one. It's especially noticeable in someone who once had a lively, active, leader-like personality.

"These are people who seem as though someone stuck a needle into their brain and removed any emotion," says geriatric psychiatrist Ken Robbins. "While they don't seem anxious, they've lost the capacity for joy."

Apathy in dementia is common: Estimates range between 50 percent and 80 percent of patients. (In contrast, only 1 percent of healthy people suffer from apathy.)

An early version of apathy looks like this: Compensating for cognitive deficits takes a great deal of attention and energy — and that creates an intense self-focus that can crowd out focus on other things, such as one's spouse or other family members, work, and outside interests. As the deficits progress, he instinctively avoids what's frustrating or consuming and pares down attention to the most critical things: remembering where he put his glasses, tying his shoes, watching a ballgame. Extraneous things — noise, visitors, questions — are tuned out.

Ultimately, it's changes to the part of the brain that handle initiation and planning — in the frontal lobes — that may be responsible, scientists think. It's a kind of impaired thinking skill known as executive function. These changes are separate from other cognitive decline and from how much emotional stress someone is under. Apathy tends to worsen as the disease progresses. What's more, those who show apathy tend to also show increased rates of cognitive decline and functional impairment, studies show.

Although some symptoms of apathy overlap with depression, they're considered distinct conditions. Someone with dementia who's depressed will also show strong emotions such as sadness, crying, hopelessness, or even suicidal thoughts. With apathy, there's just an emotional indifference.

TRY this:

- Mention symptoms of apathy to the doctor. A good psychiatric workup can be helpful in distinguishing apathy from depression. It's useful to know which you're dealing with, because someone with apathy is less likely to "snap out of it" with talk therapy and medication. Some people with apathy do improve on antidepressants, though, and some research has shown that Ritalin can boost energy and motivation.

- Avoid nagging, cajoling, and accusing. Someone who's apathetic can't help it.

- Encourage physical activity in order to keep your loved one moving, which helps overall health and mood.

- Be prepared to provide extra support with functional, everyday tasks, such as dressing, toileting, and feeding. Even if your loved one is still capable, he's likely lost the wherewithal to begin them or follow through. Step-by-step encouragement is key.

- There's some evidence that stimulating, challenging activities can improve apathy and associated depression. In one interesting 2011 study reported in the *Journal of Aging Research*, two to ten minutes of interactive, goal-driven tasks that involved physical and cognitive activity with others improved mood and quality of life, even without any improvement in executive function skills.

To help you cope:

- Remind yourself that this is a personality pattern that can be hard to deal with. Loving care, consistent routines, and encouragement can help move your loved one forward — but not always and not reliably. In other words, it IS the disease at work; it's not all up to you.

- Arrange regular respite care for yourself while someone else is keeping an eye on your loved one. An adult day center, an eldercare companion, or other sources of relief are important to your mental health. With an apathetic personality, you tend to get even less back emotionally from someone with dementia than you would in other situations. That can be incredibly depleting.

o o o

Dementia Personality Pattern: Paranoid, Frightened, and Angry

"Get rid of that one!" Astrid pointed a finger at her granddaughter Beth-Ann, who was arranging some flowers across the bedroom, helping look after her during a college break. "She's the thief! She pretends she's messing with flowers, but the minute my back is turned she'll be in my jewelry case!"

"Gran, it's me, Beth-Ann. Nobody's stealing anything!"

"So where are my pearls?" she said, accusingly, reaching up to her bare throat.

"Gran, you're in bed. Why would you have pearls on?"

Astrid only glared and shouted, "Get out!"

Beth-Ann was shaken. Her mom and dad had warned her about these outbursts. Sometimes Astrid complained about men hiding under her bed at night and robbing her the minute she fell asleep. That's why she wasn't sleeping any more, she said. She muttered to herself a lot and was obsessed about the pearl necklace she used to wear. Once she lunged at a woman in a restaurant who was wearing a similar necklace and had accused her of stealing it! When Beth-Ann's dad had tried to restrain her, she scratched at him. None of this behavior was anything like the sweet-natured Gran that Beth-Ann had grown up with.

What it looks like:

The paranoia of dementia can be baffling and deeply unnerving to families because it usually seems so out of character. But it's rooted in a strange kind of logic. Unable to comprehend what's going on — in her own head and in the everyday world around her — someone with dementia feels out of control. Things don't make sense. So her impaired thinking skills "fill in the gaps" to explain things to herself with false beliefs (called delusions). The granddaughter she fails to remember is the thief of an imagined lost necklace. The aide who wants to help give a bath becomes a would-be rapist. Night shadows are goblins, birds talk to you, crime scenes on TV shows become a window on what's happening in the next room.

As logic fails, the crippled mind of someone struggling with dementia might sense that everyone is out to harm her. These paranoid delusions are alternately frightening (which requires a lot of reassurance) or maddening (which can lead to anger and aggression).

The paranoid person with dementia may hallucinate, lash out physically, say outrageous and often cutting things, lie baldly, or show fear or mistrust.

No matter how much you try to reason or rationalize, these false thoughts can't be budged. Caregivers sometimes go to great lengths to "prove" fastidious accounting or the honesty and good record of an aide, but it's wasted effort. Logic can't cure delusions.

It's not clear how many people with dementia experience paranoia, but estimates hover around one in four.

TRY this:

- Listen empathetically and attentively, without really agreeing or disagreeing. Use neutral phrases such as, "I'm sorry you feel that way," or "That must be upsetting."

- Try deflecting the situation with a light touch if it works for the person: "Oh Gran, nobody in the world could be as beautiful as you in those pearls. Let's put them on you and you can see. I'll get a mirror."

- Sometimes it works to just wait out the moment or distract with a favorite activity, such as eating ice cream.

Tip: **"When my mom was saying crazy things, I'd make my cell phone ring and say, 'Oh, I have to take this call. Just a minute, Ma.' By the time my fake call was done, the moment would often pass." — D.R.**

- If the person becomes physical and you feel endangered, talk to the doctor. Paranoia is sometimes treated with antipsychotic medication, although this is considered a last-resort option. The FDA has warned that antipsychotics increase the risk of death in people with dementia. And although they often reduce delusions, they don't always eliminate them.

To help you cope:

- Realize that delusions are almost never rooted in any kind of reality. It's not as if Astrid always thought of her granddaughter as a sneaky type of girl and now is finally speaking the "truth." The husband who accuses his wife of infidelity likely didn't have such suspicions, or cause for such, in the whole of their marriage before the dementia. Instead, the person is reacting to something in the current reality: failure to recognize a granddaughter, a fear of being abandoned by the wife.

- Delusions also aren't rooted in anything you're doing, or not doing, in the present moment. It's not as if by caring harder or being more careful, the false thinking will disappear. The problem is rooted inside the brain.

- Get a safety net of help and support for yourself. It can be incredibly draining and toxic to listen to false accusations or live in fear of being struck. Endlessly soothing and coaxing a paranoid, fearful person can feel like you're walking on eggshells. And that's stressful. You need regular respite care, along with someone you can vent to, whether a trusted friend or a paid talk therapist or counselor. Even though you may "know" this is the disease at work, living with it can eat away at you without the reinforcement and perspective-righting help of others.

o o o

MEMORY PROBLEMS

About Memory Loss

Memory loss has become the poster symptom of Alzheimer's, even though it's far from the only effect of the disease. That's because it's particularly upsetting to the person experiencing it and frustrating to family members.

Other symptoms often appear earlier, including personality changes such as self-absorption and withdrawal, difficulty with money or math, vision trouble, and trouble finding the right words. But because memory is typically more obvious, it tends to be the first cognitive impairment symptom families notice.

A quick overview of memory loss:

The cell damage of Alzheimer's disease causes the shortest-term memories to erode first. Those that last longest tend to be very old memories (often of childhood) and emotionally rich memories (triggered by music or scent), possibly because these are stored in multiple areas of the brain.

Damage to the brain's active memory systems shows up early. Short-term memory lasts long enough to help healthy people function. It allows us to recall who just said what in a conversation, why you walked into a room, what you ate for breakfast. Even in healthy people, short-term memories tend to get crowded out by similar memories, so after a few days, it's natural to forget what you ate for breakfast three days earlier or what you wore last Saturday. It's also normal to be forgetful sometimes about what you just came into a room to do or where you parked your car. (This is often due to lack of attention.) In someone with dementia, it becomes harder to form short-term memories at all, much less to retrieve them. The person literally doesn't have short-term memories.

A type of short-term memory called working memory is also

affected. That mental "scratch pad" is where we store bits of thoughts even more briefly — the phone number we just looked up to dial, numbers used in adding a column of figures, the time just viewed on the clock. These scraps of information normally stay in our heads for a few seconds, allowing us to do something they're needed for, but then they vanish so as not to clutter the brain with unnecessary information. With dementia, these working bits also can't be held. That makes it hard to follow directions, add numbers in a checkbook, or even put on a shirt.

Short-term memory is different from long-term memory, where events have more distinction and meaning. Long-term memories are often episodic (a story, an event) or are reinforced by repetition. They're stored in multiple parts of the brain (unlike short-term memories) and can be held for a long time, even a lifetime.

Long-term memory can remain remarkably intact deep into dementia. A person who can't remember having just eaten or even own daughter might recall the names of old teachers or stories from childhood, for example.

Although memory loss plays a role in many different Alzheimer's behaviors, the following problems are among those you're most likely to encounter.

o o o

Repeats the Same Questions or Comments Within Minutes (or Less)

When Rhonda's mother first began repeating herself, Rhonda chalked it up to "old age." She tried not to be impatient when, five minutes after telling her that her cousin Sue was visiting soon, she'd ask brightly, "When are we going to see Sue again?" Her two teenagers pointed out that their Mamaw often re-told the same story about something one of her beloved pets did over and over within an hour, using the exact same words and sentences each time. "The kids were very patient, but I'd lose my marbles and yell at her, which only hurt her feelings but didn't stop the repetition," Rhonda says.

Eventually, in the evenings, Mamaw would jump up from her chair every five minutes to ask, "Have the animals been fed?"

"She was like one of those German clocks where the wooden figure pops out — only not every hour — more like every 2 minutes," Rhonda says.

WHY it happens:

A specific trigger is probably being pulled again and again: Glancing at the clock makes her wonder what time something is happening, for example. Or seeing a visiting grandchild begs the question, "So how old are you? Do you like school?" The questions and comments themselves are normal — it's the repeating that drives everyone bonkers.

Boredom or anxiety can aggravate repetition. Someone with dementia feels emotion continuously ("I don't want to be late!" or "It's my job to feed these pets!") even if she doesn't remember having just expressed the same idea.

The repetition can be a question, a comment, or an entire word-for-word anecdote.

TRY this:

At first...

- As much as you can, calmly and without comment, give the same answer. Keeping your patience is the biggest challenge.

- Try not to point out, "You just said that" or "You just asked that!" Erase phrases like, "You're not paying attention!" or "Try harder!" No matter how hard you try to get the person to see it, she literally doesn't remember having repeated herself and can't prevent it from happening again.

- Watch your body language. When you respond with sighing or eye-rolling, your loved one "reads" this emotional tone, which can make her feel anxious. The anxiety snowballs into more repetition.

If the loop persists...

- Try to identify the underlying emotion — anxiety? boredom? fear? — so you can address your comments accordingly. For example, if she sounds anxious as she's repeating something, you'd want to be extra soothing. If she just seems bored, that's a clue to engage in a fresh activity if you can.

- Use "bridge phrases" to turn the conversation in a fresh direction: "Yes, that's a funny story about Rover. *That reminds me of the time* we saw the seals at the zoo." Or, "Yes, you fed the animals. *Now why don't we* pick a TV program." Other bridge phrases: *What I'd really like to know is... I've also heard that... Yes, and did you also...* Some people respond well to being diverted to thoughts of an earlier time of life, such as childhood.

- See if you can identify a trigger that can be removed. Sometimes a particular dog dish, magazine cover, knick-knack, TV program, or other item trips a thought that gets repeated every time your loved one gazes at it. Moving or getting rid of the prompt might stop the repetition — or at least, that particular story or question. Rhonda moved the pets' feeding station out of her mother's line of vision, which finally cut down on the questions. My Dad used to read remarkable headlines aloud from the paper. Actually, it was the same headline, over and over, depending what had caught his interest. We learned to quickly swap sections whenever he'd get up to replenish his coffee, so we could hear about a different story, for a change.

- Try writing down the answer on a piece of paper: "We leave for your doctor's appointment at 2 p.m." The next time you're asked, point to the paper. Just having it in hand to look at sometimes curbs further questions.

- Find an activity that will occupy your loved one's hands and mind. This can lessen an underlying emotion causing the repetition (such as boredom or anxiety). Examples: Folding towels, matching socks, polishing silver, sorting a tool kit.

- Try moving to a different room or starting a new activity. Distraction can sometimes break the cycle.

- If she keeps asking the time, she may be finding it challenging to read a clock face. Invest in a digital clock that shows the numbers, along with the date.

To help you cope...

- Try silently counting to 10 before you answer to help calm yourself a notch. It's natural to be stressed when you're trapped in a conversational loop. Bite your lip. Do deep breathing — anything to distract yourself from reacting to the mounting frustration.

- Keeping yourself busy with a project while you talk can make the one-sided nature of the conversation slightly less frustrating.

- It's okay to leave the room for a few minutes if you feel like you'll explode. Your absence can be another form of distraction.

o o o

Forgets Recent Visits

When my grandmother could still talk on the phone, early in her dementia, our conversations would always end the same way: "So when are you coming to see me?"

It didn't matter if I had just been there the day before or an hour before. "When are you coming to see me?" she'd ask in a tone both bright and a bit plaintive.

At least I had it better than some friends, whose parents or grandparents would grow angry: "You never visit me any more!" Or (to someone who was just there in the morning and went home for lunch): "What took you so long to get here again! You act like you've forgotten all about me!" These are heartbreaking words for a family member who makes a daily visit to a loved one. — P.S.S.

WHY it happens:

Because short-term memory is shot, the encounter doesn't stick in the brain. Repetitive events also tend to run together, so one visit can seem indistinguishable from the next and is less well remembered.

It's helpful to know that, even when your recent presence has been forgotten, the mood boost of having seen you can be huge. Your loved one may not know why she feels happy (from seeing you) but she does.

TRY this:

- Instead of hearing the comment as an accusation, hear it as an expression of love. Your relative misses you and looks forward to your time together, whether you're gone for five months or five minutes.

- Gloss over the complaint: "Well, I'm here now! Let me tell you about my crazy morning." Or, "I'll visit as often as I can."

- If you're at a distance, send a calendar with the date of your next visit as a reminder.

- Take pictures at each visit, with the date. When the person complains he or she hasn't seen you lately, you can direct to a photo album to show that you have — just looking at pictures of you might be comforting.

- Vary the events at your visit. Try bringing balloons one time and a musical instrument the next. This strategy is no guarantee your outings will be better remembered, but each might stand out with more clarity.

- Whatever you do, avoid arguing. Your loved one can't follow a logical argument, and your defensiveness will only cause frustration that darkens the mood. The only relevant point is that you're there in that moment, and it should be a pleasant experience.

To help you cope:

- Try to downshift your expectations. It's not a contest of who's remembered the best. It's all about what happens in the moment.

o o o

Forgets to Take Medication (or Takes It Improperly)

One month Kara noticed that her husband ran out of some of his pills early. In addition to Aricept and Namenda, he takes a beta blocker for high blood pressure, a diuretic, an antidepressant, and several vitamins. She chalked it up to the pharmacy not giving her enough, until her pharmacist, when refilling, assured her that this was not the case. Medications are measured very carefully so that the exact dose is delivered.

The very next day, while vacuuming, she found a couple of pills under a counter near the chair where they usually took their medications in the morning, at breakfast. Maybe he was just dropping them, accidentally or on purpose, she reasoned.

That same week, her daughter Kate brought her two preschoolers over to visit. Kara was enjoying a break in the sunroom when Kate burst in. "Mom! I left the kitchen just for a minute while Dad and the kids were having breakfast together, and when I came back in, they were all excited — he was giving them his pills because they thought it was candy!" He was holding his pillbox, trying to open it, when she had walked into the room. Unsure if the kids had swallowed any (they said no and she thought not), she called Poison Control and was told what to watch for.

"They wanted some!" her dad said, when confronted. "It's good to share!"

WHY it happens:

Pill taking is both a rote task — maybe you take a vitamin every morning after brushing your teeth, without thinking about it — and a complex one. Older adults often have more than one chronic illness, involving multiple drugs that must be taken at a particular time of day, at certain intervals, with or without food, and so on. It's a lot to keep track of.

It's common to forget pills altogether, skip doses, or forget that you've already taken a medicine, and take it twice. Some pill-takers don't notice when a pill falls from the mouth. Or they don't like the taste or size of a pill and spit it out when no one's looking. As their sense of time changes, it can also be harder for them to keep track.

On top of this, people with Alzheimer's sometimes forget how certain objects are used. Pills can be mistaken for candy or as a treat or food to be shared with others.

Running out of pills early is a red flag, because it indicates that too many have been taken.

Medication mistakes are a classic early symptom of dementia that can continue and worsen. It's a sign the person can no longer manage this task independently and all aspects of handling medications must be constantly managed and monitored. It would be nice if there were an easy solution. Unfortunately, with dementia, medication management tends to rest squarely on a family member's shoulders.

TRY this:

- Make pill-taking part of the daily routine by linking it with another habit, such as drinking orange juice at breakfast or brushing teeth.

- Keep a daily log that's checked off when medications are taken, so there's a visual record.

- Also record when a prescription should be filled (or set up automatic refills), to help you track safe dosing.

- Bring the pills to the person, rather then counting on him to manage the task. Watch to make sure they're all swallowed.

- Consider telephone reminders for mild-stage impairment. Over time, this isn't a reliable way to monitor. You'll need a visual check, actually seeing the person swallow the pill. To find a reminder service, enter *telephone medication reminder* in a search engine.

For safer dispensing:

- Switch to a day-of-the-week pill dispenser if you don't already use one. There are also versions for a.m./ p.m. Some versions lock or have self-timers or alarms, which can help someone early in the disease who's living independently.

- Look into high-tech dispensers. This landscape is changing fast, and there are many options; search online for what's available. Some send a text or email reminder; others tie into companies, so that if a pillbox isn't opened by a certain time, a call is triggered. *It's really important to realize, however, that these methods only work in the earliest stages, and then only for some people.* New gadgets are difficult for people with cognitive impairment to master. Often the dispensers' real value is when a message or alert is sent as a reminder to you, the caregiver.

- Get help getting started. Pill dispensers only work well if they're properly filled in the first place. A 2011 Northwestern University study found that 60 percent of paid caregivers made errors when sorting meds into pillboxes. Ask the pharmacist to do it for you when prescriptions are filled. Some will do this routinely; others will do it once or twice to show you how. It can be confounding to figure out what "three times a day" or "every eight hours" looks like in the compartments of a pill organizer. After you get help the first time, draw yourself a "map" of the pills' look and name and where each goes.

- Fill dispensers at a quiet time when you're feeling alert. It's not a multitasking kind of job.

Tip: **"Our pharmacist dispensed the pills in blister packs, so you could see if one was taken or not. We'd write the date on the pack above each pill on the pack." — S. K.**

More safety tips:

- Make sure you understand what each drug is used for

and the proper dosing schedule, as well as possible side effects to watch for (especially for a new medication).

- Keep a master list of medications in two places: on your refrigerator or other central location and in your wallet, so you have it handy at doctor visits. In the event of a hospitalization or specialist appointment, you might be the only person with the complete drug picture.

- Lock up or store out of reach all extra medications, as well as other household members' prescriptions, so nothing gets mixed up or taken out of turn. "Out of sight, out of mind" is a good rule of thumb to avoid tempting your loved one into self-medicating out of turn.

- Bring all prescription drugs, supplements, and over-the-counter medications used regularly (such as OTC drugs for pain or constipation), in their original containers, to the next primary-care checkup. Ask the doctor for a medication review to assess whether each is needed. The fewer meds taken, the fewer to be remembered — and the fewer mistakes or side effects you're likely to encounter.

- For someone who tends to balk at taking pills, offer an incentive, such as ice cream afterward. Pick a time of day when your loved one is most agreeable or well rested, if possible.

- Check to make sure no pills are too big to be comfortably swallowed. if so, check with the doctor and/or pharmacist about more manageable alternatives. Some medications can be dispensed in liquid form and then mixed with other foods.

o o o

Forgets to Turn Off Stove

The smell of gas hit Jason as soon as he opened the door to his grandparents' house. His first thought was that there was a leak, and he was about to call the gas company. Once in the kitchen, though, he saw the stove burner on, blue-orange gas flames flicking into the air, with no pot or other sign of cooking in sight.

He quickly turned the burner off, noticing blackened marks around the knobs from previous burns, and opened some windows.

His grandparents were sitting obliviously in the living room, watching TV.

WHY it happens:

Forgetting to turn off the stove can happen to anyone as a result of inattention and preoccupation. Toss in progressive memory loss, and it's a recipe for kitchen danger.

Some people with mild impairment can manage on their own for a while longer, with some safety checks in place. But the inability to use a stove safely or cook is a red flag for being unable to live independently.

TRY this:

- Consider unplugging a stove and plugging it in only when someone capable is using it. Make sure the plug can't be seen by the person with dementia, who many not notice what you've done. Another option is to use the shut-off valve (gas stove) or circuit breaker (electric stove).

- Keep a microwave and electric teakettle for use by the person with dementia. Prepare meals in advance, and put them in separate containers so a single meal's serving can be heated up. A hot water dispenser can be an easy way to provide hot water for soup, tea, or coffee, but it can also be a burn risk. (Older skin is more fragile.)

- If you can afford it, look for a replacement stove that has automatic shut-off after a certain period of time. Timers and motion sensors that detect activity around the stove help prevent accidents.

- Remove the knobs, so the stove can't be turned on.

- To make sure your loved one is getting essential nutrition, look into home delivery of meals, through programs such as Meals on Wheels.

o o o

Gets Lost When Driving

Norm liked to drive, and even though his memory problems were getting worse, he seemed to manage a car just fine. One Saturday, he and his wife, Elaine, were out for their usual drive to the farmer's market on the edge of town.

"Norm! You missed the turn!"

Norm looked unconcerned. "We'll just go another way," he said.

Elaine settled back in her seat. After five or 10 minutes, she realized they weren't traveling anywhere near the farmer's market. "Norm, where are we?"

He didn't answer.

"Are you sure this road goes there?"

"I know a shortcut," he said confidently.

After another few minutes, Elaine realized she had no idea where they were and seemed to be traveling in the wrong direction. "But how do we get to the farmer's market from over here?" she persisted.

"Oh, is that where you want to go?" Norm said. "Is it today?"

Elaine then realized that Norm must have forgotten the way well before the first missed turn and they'd been driving aimlessly all this time.

WHY it happens:

Some people with memory loss do well on familiar routes for a while. Even so, there usually comes a day when they miss a turn or lose track of where they were heading. And you can't quite be sure when that day will come. A report on 207 lost drivers with dementia, in the *American Journal of Occupational Therapy*, points out just how dangerous this can be. Only 116 of the lost drivers were found alive, and about a third of those were injured. In another study of 106 drivers with dementia — mostly men in their 50s to 90s who lived with a caregiver — the majority were on routine errands close to home when they became lost. One in ten were found in a different state!

Backtracking is a complicated cognitive process. Usually the person tends to just keep going — sometimes realizing the error and hoping to see a familiar landmark, sometimes just continuing obliviously. (Sometimes both!)

TRY this:

- If your loved one is missing while driving, contact local law enforcement immediately. Don't wait several hours to see if he turns up. Most missing older drivers are located by the police. If your state has a Silver Alert system, it can be lifesaving.

- If it happens just once, with a safe outcome, thank your lucky stars and consider it a wake-up call that your loved one can no longer drive safely. Not only his life, but the lives of others on the road or walking and bicycling on the streets are at risk. It's time to take steps to keep your loved one from driving, and come up with viable alternatives.

o o o

Forgets Someone Died

On the morning after my mother died, after a very short illness, in a hospital bed placed by home hospice in the living room of the house where I grew up, my four siblings and I sat together in the kitchen, our dumbfounded shock still raw. We heard the stairs creak as Dad came down — dressed in a suit. Grim and businesslike, he was ready to go to the funeral home to make arrangements. He often forgot appointments or what he'd just said, but he remembered this important mission. Despite his advancing dementia, he seemed almost like his old self, or at least a grief-stricken version of his usual sunny self.

The next morning, the scene was repeated. Numb siblings, whispered funeral plans over breakfast, and then Dad's footfalls on the staircase. "Good morning," he said in a bright voice. "Are you ready to go see Mother at the hospital?"

"Go see her?"

"She's doing well and sends her love to all of you."

My sisters and I exchanged uneasy glances. "Dad, Mom died two days ago. Remember?"

He burst into tears, stricken anew. "Why didn't anybody tell me? I didn't get to say goodbye!" — P.S.S.

WHY it happens:

This is an extreme yet typical example. Often people with dementia can't remember a death that happened more distantly. They may express an interest in talking to someone who died years ago, such as a parent. They may be uncertain about the death of a close family member: "Did my brother Bill die?" Or they may be oblivious — for example, talking about inviting Joan and Ralph over to dinner, when Joan or Ralph (or both) died some time ago.

Psychologists have told me that my father (who was deep in middle-stage dementia at the time) was able to recall, the next morning, that his wife had died because the shock of this seismic event was so great. But as time wore on — in this case, less than 48 hours — days ran together and the fact of her death grew less distinct and more easily forgotten. Actually it's hard to say whether Dad continued to remember the day of her death in more than a general way. After the funeral, he never mentioned my mother (to whom he was married for 67 years and never left the house without kissing) to us again.

TRY this:

- Gently orient the person when he brings it up: "Dad, Mom died two days ago." "I'm sorry, Joan was killed in a car crash in 1988."

- Expect to hear an expression of grief, crying, or other response. That's a normal human response. There's no harm in this; it's not going to make their Alzheimer's any better or worse. Respond with the same empathy and love as you would whether it was new grief or a fresh rekindling of grief.

- Brace yourself for no response. Some people, reminded of a death, say things like, "Oh." Or, "I sure do miss her" and then leave it at that. Or they may say nothing. Don't misconstrue these responses to mean that your loved one didn't love the person. The response given may be all he's capable of right now. It's okay.

- Turn the fact of the death into an opportunity for fond reminiscing: "Wasn't she the sweetest person ever?" "I'll always miss her piano playing. I remember the time she gave that concert at the school…."

- Don't make a big deal about insisting the person absorb the reality (driving him to a cemetery to "prove" the death, showing an obituary, etc.). Some people will ask follow-up questions, and others will be accepting and not talk about it further.

- Consider distraction if he becomes fixated on contacting some long-gone relative or wants to buy things for her and can't seem to process the reality of a death.

- Ultimately, decide what's best in your particular case. Some families find it easier to tell a little white lie when the questioning is persistent or the person becomes quite agitated every time the topic comes up. It's possible to gloss over the fact, especially as dementia advances. When one woman kept asking about her long-dead husband, her daughter and son would put her off by saying, "He's running late." Or, "He's still on that trip to China" (where their dad in fact once traveled for business). Such comments would pacify her in the moment, and then she'd forget about it. This is a less-good strategy, of course, if your loved one fixates on this falsehood and waits around all day in disappointment.

Should You Tell Someone With Dementia About a Death?

Many families often also wonder whether to inform someone with dementia of the death of a loved one in the first place. The rationale people give for not saying anything is usually to avoid causing unnecessary distress. Some caregivers say they avoid sharing sad news because they don't want to be asked about it (and have to talk about it or revisit their own grief) over and over.

Most dementia experts agree, though, that the better approach is to be candid. Everyone has a right to know this information, regardless of mental state.

Yes, he or she may have a strong emotional reaction. That's okay. Seeing a household grieving without being told why is also something the person can pick up on and become distressed by. In a nutshell, it's almost always better to know — even if the information is quickly forgotten.

Geri Hall, a wonderful memory-care expert and nurse who has worked at the University of Iowa and the Banner Alzheimer's Institute in Arizona, offers some good advice:

- Tell the person at a time of day that tends to be best for him. Morning? After a meal?

- Make sure the place is free of distractions — TV and radio off, no crowds around.

- It's okay to show emotion yourself. Take the person's hand.

- Establish the context for who you're talking about. Don't make it like a quiz: "Do you remember Jack?" But help make clear whom you're talking about.

- Don't be surprised if the person with Alzheimer's reacts by trying to comfort you. Some people, depending on their faith, culture, and personal mobility, welcome attending a funeral.

"Think about it," Hall says. "If it were you who had dementia, wouldn't you want to know if your loved one had passed?"

o o o

Distorted Sense of Time

In the house where I grew up, the laundry was located in the basement. When my mom would go down to throw in a load, my dad (now with dementia) would quickly grow upset. He'd walk to the top of the stairs and shout down, "What are you doing down there?"

"Laundry!" she'd reply.

A few minutes would pass. He'd go back to the top of the stairs, and slowly make his way down them.

"What?" she'd say.

"I was looking for you," he'd reply.

"I just told you, I was throwing in some wash!"

Conversely, when my Dad went down to the laundry, maybe taking a load from the washer to the dryer, he could be gone for a full hour. Then it was my mom who'd grow curious and creep to the top of the stairs: "Pat! What are you doing down there?" He could fold towels for ages. — P.S.S.

WHY it happens:

Cognitive changes distort the ability to keep track of time. An hour can seem like five minutes. Five minutes can seem like an hour.

TRY this:

- Be patient. Your loved one might ask you repeatedly, "What time is it?" or might grow anxious or clingy if you leave the room or are out of sight for several minutes.

- Know that it's futile to argue or say things like, "But we just got here!" or, "I was only gone for two minutes."

- Make sure clocks are visible in every room your loved one frequents. Digital clocks are usually easier to read. This may temporarily reduce anxiety early in dementia.

My dad, for example, checked his watch constantly deep into moderate-stage dementia; it seemed to reassure him. But eventually it will grow harder for your loved one to track passing time.

- Try setting a timer when you have to leave the room — to go do laundry in the basement, for example. "I'll be back in ten minutes," you might say, "when the bell rings." When you return, be sure to make your presence known. If you do this often, the person gets used to the idea of the bell as a time cue, and may sit patiently by the ticking timer awaiting your return. An old-fashioned hourglass timer that lasts a few minutes works, too.

- Try to always be prompt or early — don't stay away or out of sight longer than you said you would. Announce your return.

- Check in periodically when you're both around the house, so you're not out of sight for too long.

- Keep a large calendar in a central area where you can record appointments. Review it in the morning (and as needed through the day) to reassure your loved one that he won't miss any important events.

- Try to stretch out the visit with a distraction when you're out in public and the person insists, after just five minutes, "I want to go home." You can say, "Just a few more minutes . . . we're about to hear some music/look at some pictures/have some coffee." Realize, though, that if he grows more agitated, the simplest course may be to leave and try again another day.

- Structure the day around a solid routine. The predictable flow of activities — meals, a walk, TV time, nap, so on — will help the person mark time during the day.

o o o

Doesn't Recognize Familiar People

Toward the end of his life, my father was living in a nursing home for rehabilitation following a small stroke. At every visit, he'd reach for a copy of Woman's Day magazine, which he kept on his bedside table. For years, I'd been a columnist for the magazine, writing about family.

He'd hand me the magazine, pointing to my picture on a carefully bookmarked page. "Have you read Paula's new article?"

He knew I was familiar. He knew, I'm pretty sure, that I was family. But which family, exactly, had grown muddled. He often introduced me to the nursing staff (who knew me) as "my sister" or "my sister Betty." But then he would ask after my children, sometimes by name.

There's nothing quite like the astonishment that grabs you the first time this person you've known your entire life, including just the day before, can't quite place you. I felt an odd mix of understanding and disbelief.

Dad always seemed to know I was a person who loved him, and — for both of us — that had to be enough. — P.S.S.

WHY it happens:

The inability to recognize friends and family — even a spouse or adult child — is a byproduct of declining memory.

Often it's a matter of "last to know, first to go." Those who entered the person's life later, including grandchildren, sons- or daughters-in-laws, some colleagues — tend to be forgotten before siblings, for example. Names tend to slip first. (My Dad often asked, "How's the family?" to cover for the fact that he wasn't sure which of us had children and who they were.) Your loved one may know that a certain face is familiar without being able to state the exact relationship.

Familiar people get confused with others, too. It's common for an adult daughter to be mistaken for a wife, for example — even to the point of the father making advances.

It's important to understand what are NOT reasons for this confusion: You're not forgotten because you weren't around enough, or emotionally close enough, or because you aren't loving or giving enough now. Being forgotten or confused for another isn't a reflection on you or the quality of your relationship.

TRY this:

- At first, gently offer the correct name or relationship, if you like: "Actually I'm Paula, his daughter. You've always said I look like Betty, haven't you, Dad?" I'd say to the staff after being wrongly introduced. Or I'd say "Dad" a lot to re-orient him. Just try to do it in a way that preserves your loved one's dignity.

- Ultimately, you have to let it pass. If he keeps forgetting or truly seems to have no idea who you are, let it go. ("Yup, I've read all her articles," I'd say of the magazine columnist Paula, a.k.a. me.) It doesn't really matter.

- Pre-empt trouble by offering a prompt when you see him: "Hi, Dad, it's Paula, your favorite middle daughter!" "Look who's come to see you, your old bowling buddy Norm!"

- Forewarn friends or those who haven't seen him in awhile, so they're prepared.

- Avoid turning it into a test. My dad (before his dementia was obvious) used to quiz his mother-in-law, who had Alzheimer's and knew no one by the end: "Do you know me? How about her — do you know who this is?" That puts unnecessary stress on the person with memory loss. (My dad, who had little knowledge about dementia, seemed truly befuddled that she could forget everyone.)

- If your loved one behaves inappropriately — for example, a father making a pass at a daughter — avoid blowing it out of proportion. Remember the "why." Instead, stay calm and distract the person, then redirect the behavior to something else. "I have an idea, let's go get some chocolate." "I'm tired, how about a walk in the fresh air?"

To help you cope:

- Realize that your presence is registered and matters! People sometimes think, "Why should I bother visiting? He doesn't even know me." But even after names and relations are lost to the person, close relationships still register as beloved, familiar figures. Your presence is cheering, comforting, and de-stressing. A rose is still a rose, and smells as sweet, even if you don't know what that pretty pink fragrant thing that cheers you up is called.

o o o

HELP-RELATED ISSUES

Resists Seeing a Doctor

The whispers among M.J.'s family members grew more urgent: What's up with Mom? Have you noticed? M.J., who lived half a mile away, was the first to notice. Her two sisters across the state finally agreed they couldn't ignore the funny behaviors any more — how Mom mixed up two grandchildren's names, the day Mom had her second fender bender in a week, the time she showed up for a family dinner but had the day wrong.

"Mom, you feeling okay?" they'd ask.

"I'm fine. Your poor old ma is just getting older," Adele, their mother, would say.

Then she knocked over her daughter's mailbox while backing down the drive, during a visit in which she'd forgotten the year her husband died, and the cookies she'd made were oddly inedible. All small things? M.J., a nurse, knew otherwise.

The girls sat her down together to insist she get checked out. Adele flatly denied there was a problem. She blamed the car accident on the weather (as she had the previous two incidents) and the cookies on "a bad batch of flour." If ever she acknowledged a misstep at all (she often didn't), there was always an excuse — a headache, a lousy receptionist, bad drivers, and her favorite, "You misheard me."

WHY it happens:

Someone having problems might resist seeing a doctor due to:

- Dread: She suspects a brain-related illness, but the stigma of Alzheimer's is enough to make her play ostrich and ignore it. (That's likely, since Alzheimer's is the second most feared disease, after cancer.)

- Procrastination: She's aware that she's making mistakes and having trouble with thinking skills but hopes the problem will clear up and go away.

- Denial: She truly doesn't see it as a problem that merits a doctor's attention — the "just old age" rationale.

- Dislike of medical care: She avoids doctors generally.

- Obliviousness. Her case is advanced to the point where she fails to recognize a problem.

To all this, add the complexities of other people in your life telling you what you "should" do (get to a doctor). When the message comes from adult children, a parent may feel it's "not your business." Even when the message comes from a spouse, there can be a resistance borne in dread, that the person you trust most is confirming your deepest fear. And some prickly personality types perceive any suggestions as nagging.

Most cases of dementia of all kinds actually go undiagnosed, says the U.S. Preventive Services Task Force. Mostly, this is because people don't get screened or evaluated in the first place. Usually aware of a problem at first, they avoid the doctor or don't take symptoms seriously. Family members, too, can get in the way of a health evaluation. A 2012 study by the Alzheimer's Foundation of America found that two-thirds of those who saw behavioral symptoms of Alzheimer's in a loved one felt they were "just a normal part of aging." (They weren't.) Of these, 67 percent said that such thinking delayed getting a diagnosis.

Sometimes doctors miss the signs because the person pulls it together for the duration of the exam. In one small study from 2000, 11 in 14 people found to have mild dementia had no record of it in their medical charts; nor did five in seven of those with moderate dementia or one in five with severe dementia.

With today's improved screenings, doctors can make a probable diagnosis of Alzheimer's with as much as 90 percent certainty.

TRY this:

- **Start by believing in the benefits of early diagnosis.** What's the big deal about putting a name to the problem? Does it matter if you know the exact reason Mom is forgetful or Dad gets lost driving? As with any health matter, it's best to know exactly what you're dealing with. Memory loss, poor judgment, and other symptoms aren't natural byproducts of getting older. Nor do they necessarily mean Alzheimer's. Many conditions mimic Alzheimer's. By having a professional opinion on what's normal or not, you can get reversible problems treated. The latter include depression, medication reactions or dosage problems, and a condition called normal pressure hydrocephalus (caused when cerebrospinal fluid collects in the brain) — all curable.

And if it is Alzheimer's or another form of dementia? (Many times there's a mix of causes, including vascular dementia caused by small strokes.) Starting lifestyle changes and treatments sooner, including medications, rather than later, can slow impairment. Knowing what you're dealing with gives you a chance to learn about the course of the disease, so you're not always blindsided. An early diagnosis can make your loved one eligible for, and able to benefit from, clinical trials. You can also find out about community resources. And knowing early gives your loved one a valuable chance to have input on important decisions before it's too late.

It's true that you don't need an official diagnosis or label to help the person manage daily life with dementia. The issues you deal with will mostly be the same. But most caregivers find the path easier when they know for sure what they're dealing with.

- **Respect what the person having symptoms might be feeling.** Denial is a powerful and self-protective emotion. That's why many people prefer to ignore bothersome symptoms rather than risk having to confront a problem. Some people fear the stigma that Alzheimer's still carries, especially in some cultures.

Fear feeds denial. It's helpful to reassure: You're safe and you're with me, no matter what. We'll figure it out.

Try appealing to the brighter side: Remind her that there are many different causes of memory loss and other cognitive symptoms, besides Alzheimer's, and most can be treated. If it is Alzheimer's, nothing will change overnight. She'll still be the same person who walked into the doctor's office. But now you'll know what you're up against and can do something about it.

- **Pursue diagnosis on a timetable that makes sense.** If you're still met with resistance, tread lightly. While you're smart to stick with your resolve to have concerns checked out, you have to realize that you might need to slow down. Badgering or bickering about it tends to lead to more resistance. It's best to tread with compassion. The reality is that how you proceed from day to day isn't likely to change much whether you have a confirmed diagnosis of Alzheimer's or not.

There's usually no rush. As symptoms progress, she may be more willing to see a doctor, or a regular exam will come up for another reason. You can call in your concerns in advance of the appointment.

- **Create a record.** It's almost always family members, more than physicians, who spot the first signs of Alzheimer's disease. Write down examples of what you and others are seeing. You'll be better able to notice patterns or changes in the frequency of certain behaviors than you would by keeping a mental record. This evidence is incredibly useful when you speak with medical professionals and may help when discussing the topic with family and friends.

Write down:

- Examples of memory loss

- Specific safety incidents (car accident, falls, getting lost, stove burners left on, etc.)

- Other unusual behaviors (incontinence, out-of-character outbursts, mood swings, etc.)

The key is change: anything that's different for that individual. Be sure to note when you first noticed a particular change in behavior, physical ability, or mental ability (or about how long the change has been occurring); how frequently it occurs; if it has worsened; and how unlike the person it is.

This same notebook can also serve as your "playbook" throughout your family's journey, a central source of all the information that will be needed not only to make a diagnosis, but to formulate an ongoing care plan. Having all the information you need in one place can be a valuable shortcut for families.

What else to record:

- Any current and past medical problems and conditions

- Current medications and their dosages

- Other family members' histories of illnesses (especially diabetes and Alzheimer's disease and other types of dementia)

- Contact information for doctors and pharmacists

- A record of who has been consulted and when

Learn a bit more about Alzheimer's. While you're dealing with resistance, invest a little time in getting more familiar with the disease. Having a basic understanding allows you to ask doctors more informed questions and recognize the signs to watch for.

Creative solutions:

- Try a "side door" approach to getting your loved one to a doctor. Make it about you: "I know you feel perfectly healthy, but I've heard everyone over 60 should see the doctor once a year to check the heart and blood sugar and you'll help me sleep better if you do that." If you're worried about one parent, get both parents to agree to "get checked out."

- Try a third-party approach. Sometimes spouses or parents won't listen to us but will willingly follow the suggestions of a friend, clergyperson, or other relative with more distance and less emotional history.

- Register your concerns with the person's primary care doctor. You can do this even if you don't have legal access to her health records. The doctor can't release information to you without the patient's consent, but you can share information or concerns. Ideally, time your call for just before a scheduled exam.

Really creative solutions:

- Appeal to pride. Some people might be persuaded to consult a specialist if you highlight something truly "special" about it to them: "This clinic is where so-and-so celebrity / local elites all go." Lisa P. Gwyther and Dr. Murali Doraiswamy, in their _Alzheimer's Action Plan_, note that this tactic got one women to see a specialist with a "Christian medical practice," and another man agreed to a certain institution because it had once "saved my father's life." A former academic might be persuaded by an article about the doctor or clinic you have in mind.

- Try a little white lie: "The insurance company says you have to have a physical."

- Try getting a family member to the doctor for an entirely different reason — a follow-up exam for a chronic condition, an unrelated symptom. Beforehand, express your concerns about memory, cognition, and other issues so the doctor is on alert. In the absence of another reason for an exam, consider asking the doctor about inviting your relative in for a checkup on some other pretext (a flu shot, an overdue preventative test); some may agree to this in order to check out your concerns.

- Look into house calls. Some physicians, gerontologists, and geriatric care managers are among those who provide them and can do an initial assessment.

- Attend a free screening during the National Memory Screening Day, usually held in November, sponsored by the Alzheimer's Foundation of America. This may appeal to the budget-minded.

- Pitch prevention, without mentioning your suspicions: "I hear there's a lot we can do now to avoid Alzheimer's and memory problems — let's find out what we can both do." Or, "Let's all go to get a baseline screening about how our brains are working now — then we can go have lunch after."

o o o

Rebuffs Your Assistance

"Certain subjects in our house were just taboo," recalls Kate. "And as my parents got older, #1 was the subject of their getting older. It just wasn't mentioned."

This drove Kate's husband, Dave, crazy. In his family, everybody talked about everything. His widowed mother was very open to Dave and his brothers taking care of her lawn, her house, and her finances.

Not so Kate's father. By the time his wife died, the house was already in disrepair. Two family inheritances had left the attics and hallways of the old house cluttered with extra furniture. He didn't cook much, either — which Kate secretly thought of as a blessing because she was afraid he might start a fire (even as she worried about his diet). He clearly needed help — but he carried on as if he were still 60 and hale, and besides, he said, it was "none of her damn beeswax."

"You have to do something!" Dave would say after each visit or crisis.

To which Kate would always say, "Yeah, but what? How?"

WHY it happens:

To allow help is to admit you need help. The number-one reason older adults often refuse assistance is *fear of losing control.* (It's number two and three and four, too.) Maintaining control is one of the driving needs of an older adult from the perspective of human development, says geriatric psychology and communication expert David Soulie. "Each day, they feel losses — of strength, health, peers, and authority — that are staggering," he writes in his insightful book, *How to Say It to Seniors.*

Other factors that may contribute:

- *Pride and dignity.* Cooking, maintaining a home, or other aspects of self-care are a point of pride for many. They see any intimation that they're no longer up to the task as insulting.

- *Stoicism.* Some people adapt to their "lot" in life, whatever it is. They had tough times before and see their current challenges as tough times to weather again.

- *Fractious relationships.* Resistance can be higher when there's suspicion (founded or not) of a family member's motives, such as concerns over money or a history of discord. Someone who doesn't believe you have his best interests at heart will balk.

- *Lack of insight.* In the early stages of Alzheimer's, your loved one may recognize that he's not managing as well but resist help. As the disease progresses beyond a certain point, he'll eventually lack the ability to recognize that there's a problem.

The problem of a parent refusing help is among the most common and frustrating adult children encounter. Inserting yourself into someone's life is a worthy goal when you're doing it for his own benefit. But parents don't always see it that way. They're driven by a need for control, and we're driven by a need to solve problems, get things done, tick items off a to-do list, and move forward. That disconnect can be crazymaking — for both sides.

Someone with dementia is still a person with free will and preferences that deserve to be respected — up to the point when safety becomes an issue.

Knowing when you've reached that point, though, is never easy.

Early in the disease, people can often continue to live independently but with an ever-increasing need for support. That's when you want to tread carefully and compassionately, while exploring creative strategies for providing any necessary help. At the same time, you have to constantly monitor your loved one's environment to keep him safe from his own limitations and from external threats — everything from financial scammers and getting lost to malnourishment when he can no longer cook. You have a moral duty to keep those around him safe, too, from being run down by his poor driving or burned out of their apartment building because he forgot to turn off a burner. This part of the journey can be a tricky dance, depending on the tone of your relationship and your loved one's personality, among other factors.

Eventually, everyone with Alzheimer's, if they live long enough, will need help in most areas of life. It becomes unsafe or impossible to do almost anything without supervision or help. If you're not at that point yet, it will come. That's when the tricky dance can become downright unpleasant, because you have to assert yourself in ways that may feel unnatural or unkind. And it can be hard to know when you've shifted from one phase to the next, because there's generally a long gray zone in the middle.

TRY this:

In the beginning....

- Understand what "no" means. Soulie points out that knee-jerk refusals often come from the older person's compelling need to maintain control. It's a natural response to the conflicts they're feeling: coping with so many losses and threats, as well as to anyone (family caregivers included) trying to meddle and create more changes. Having empathy for this perspective can guide your communication. Let your loved one know that you get where he's coming from.

- Listen more than you act, at first. Your goal is to help, not fight about the need for help. Invest time nurturing a relationship on a neutral, rather than adversarial, track. Spend time together not with the aim of nagging or saying what you think should be done but just relaxing and listening. Reassure him that you care about his perspective. You'll be able to achieve more if he doesn't feel like you're "taking over" or "intruding."

- Observe and record what you're dealing with. It can help to get specific about where you see help is needed. Make written lists of the problems (bill collectors are calling about unpaid bills, three car accidents, can't mow lawn, got lost last week, etc.). Ask others in the person's world, such as old friends and neighbors, if they've noticed anything amiss. There's no shame in saying, "Hey, I'm worried about Dad, and I wonder if he's seemed his usual self to you?"

- Also, carefully research solutions before bringing them up. What resources are available in your community? Call the local Area Agency on Aging, which is a great starting point that will direct you to programs and services for specific needs. Your local Alzheimer's Association chapter may also have a list of services. If the problem is driving, what are alternate ways he could get around (paratransit? relatives pitching in to drive?). If the problem is home repair, who can do it? If you need a nursing aide, what are the reputable services in town? Should you hire from them or try to find someone independently, which is usually cheaper but not regulated? Ask friends and colleagues. If you work for a large company, ask your human resources department for ideas.

- Talk about the need for help only when your loved one is relaxed and in a good mood. Consider whether you're the best messenger. Maybe a discussion about help would be more effective coming from the looked-up-to eldest sibling, a family friend, or a trusted doctor.

- Instead of making suggestions, ask questions: "I know you don't want to move, but how do you think we should handle upkeep on the house now that the doctor says you can't go up ladders?" "What do you want to do with all this extra stuff in the house?" "Why don't you make a list of pros and cons?" "What's the most difficult part of living alone for you?"

Try to listen for an underlying reason behind resistance that you might be able to address: concern about money or dislike of something new, for example. *I used to think grab bars were ugly things, but I was reading up on what's called universal design, and now they're this trendy thing everyone wants and might help improve the value of the house. Or, this program at the center is free if you're over 65 — that's why Carol's mom and her friends all started going.*

- Keep focused on the solution and the benefits. *If someone helps with cleaning, I'll have more time to take you to lunch and the salon. When your meals are brought to you, I won't have to worry as much, and you'll get your energy back.*

- Watch your language. Some people bristle at certain words, like "help," notes Carol D. O'Dell, a caregiving consultant who looked after her own mother for many years. Maybe *assistance* will be more readily accepted, she suggests. Try words like *maid service* if "cleaners" offends, or *car service* instead of "somebody to drive you around."

- Propose "temporary" solutions: *Why don't you try this for a couple of months and see how it goes for you? The firm offers a trial service for a month. The first visit is free, so what's there to lose?* One caregiver persuaded her parents to have a geriatric care manager (who was referred to as a *life coach*) drop by daily while she was out of town. Her parents enjoyed the help so much that the arrangement continued after the daughter's business trip ended.

- Do what you can to prevent possible problems. Often there are things you can do without your loved one's permission or awareness that can extend his ability to live independently. You can turn down the temperature of the hot water to avoid accidental scalding, for example, or stop magazine subscriptions that pile up unread and get tripped over.

Creative solutions:

- Mask the purpose of the help. Caregivers have hit on many clever strategies to bring in help, based on the quirks of their loved one and the needs of the situation. To help keep an eye on her mother across the country, for example, attorney and consumer advocate Barbara

Kate Repa enlisted local friends who stopped by on pretexts. One friend asked Repa's mother to save the newspaper for her because she didn't subscribe; every day or so she'd drop by to collect them. Another friend asked for knitting lessons. She also got her mom to accept Meals on Wheels services by telling her she was "rating" them for a work assignment and needed her help evaluating them.

- Bestow a gift. Your mother might not like the idea of a cook and maid because she's old and needs help, but she might get a kick out of a birthday gift for these services pitched as "pampering."

- Find the right inroad. Someone who never hired help but always follows clergy or medical advice might be open to someone coming in if recommended by the right person. Someone who grew up with household help might be more open to it, freeing you up to handle the caregiving chores.

- Invoke others. Some people are more accepting if they know it's what their peers do: "Jane's parents have a maid now" (even if that person is actually a personal aide).

- Know your audience. Some people are swayed by exclusivity or impressive credentials: "This is the best geriatric care manager in town, Mom." "It usually takes six months to get an appointment with this lawyer, but she had a cancellation and can see you next week."

- Keep in mind that it's hard to force anybody to do anything. You may have to live with decisions or living situations you're not thrilled with and wait for the proverbial other shoe to drop. This can be agonizing, especially as the effects of dementia begin to take hold. You may be only able to do what you can preventatively, until things reach the point where finances, health, or physical safety are in jeopardy.

When safety is at risk....

Sometimes families successfully get together and intervene to protect a loved one in danger. This tends to work better with a married couple. At first both refuse help, but as the dementia worsens, the well spouse capitulates and agrees that a new situation demands changes. Or in the case of a single parent, he may decline to the point where family members are simply able to take on more and more, with less and less resistance.

What if these options don't pan out? You have plenty of company. Many families are driven to wit's end over this issue. If help is refused and your family member continues to act in irresponsible or dangerous ways, you may have to resort to the "big gun" of the law.

- If he has previously assigned powers of attorney for health care and finances, it may be time to invoke those documents. Often this is a matter of a doctor or designated others declaring that the person can't make the relevant decisions.

- If you don't already have legal authority, you may need to seek adult guardianship, a more complex maneuver. It's also known as "conservatorship" in some states. You'll have to petition a judge to declare that the person is unable to make major decisions for himself and has made no previous documentation for what should happen in this event. The same person, or two different people, might be assigned to manage health decisions and financial-legal decisions.

  The benefits are huge: Your family gets clarity in a dangerous and disintegrating situation about how to safeguard your loved one.

  Unfortunately, guardianship is an expensive and often fraught process. You have to hire a lawyer and go before a judge. If your loved one still has some awareness (or good days and bad, where it comes and goes), he can feel humiliated or emotionally manipulate the very family members who are trying to save him. And when families disagree over who should handle decision-making, a mediator may also need to be involved.

If you go this route, look for an attorney who specializes in elder law. You'll need someone experienced to walk you through the nuances and help you prepare a case in an expedient way. You may have heard that it's difficult to obtain adult guardianship, but in cases of Alzheimer's, it tends to be much easier to prove the need for this step.

To help you cope:

- Try not to get caught up in thoughts like these: "I don't want to hurt her feelings." "That would be insulting to her dignity." "She'll hate me if I do that." "That's just not done in our family." Such beliefs might be true in a perfect world, but once your loved one has advancing dementia, you're in Alzheimer's world. To keep someone safe, the need for safety has to trump convention, pride, and hurt feelings. It's hard, but it's true.

- Don't take these clashes personally. It's not about you, the wisdom of your insights, the kindness of your heart, or the brilliance of your solutions. Recalcitrance has everything to do, instead, with the affected person's motivations and place in life. You might not get anywhere faster by taking your emotions out of the equation, but you'll get there calmer and with a better relationship.

o o o

BEHAVIOR PROBLEMS

Aggression (Acting Hostile or Violent)

"Carl didn't have a mean bone in his body," his widow, Esther, recalls. "He was as gentle as you can imagine helping birth a stuck foal or holding a grandbaby or oh, just anything."

Alzheimer's disease changed Carl. Though never a big talker, he became taciturn and sometimes even rude. He'd say curt, cutting things to visitors. He'd turn and leave the room on them. To Esther, his wife of 57 years, he was mostly docile and polite. Until the "ham sandwich incident," that is.

"I was serving him a late lunch one afternoon because we'd been out at the market," she says. "And when I put the ham sandwich down in front of him, he looked at it like he didn't know what it was, so I told him. 'I don't like ham! You know that!' he bellowed at me. I was so surprised.

"'Why Carl, of course you do,' I told him, easy as you please. And he reached up and slapped me across the face!" Esther is as astonished today, telling that story, as she was four years ago when it happened. "He'd never raised a hand to me for the world!"

That day marked a turning point. Carl continued to react with a raised hand whenever he didn't like something or didn't want to do it. Sometimes he grabbed her by the arm and clenched it. Esther, a petite woman, grew afraid. She hid Carl's rough behavior from her son until he saw it firsthand and made the connection to the bruises his mother had been making excuses for. They were investigating nursing homes when Carl died of a stroke.

WHY it happens:

Lashing out is usually a result of both brain changes and environmental factors. It's extremely upsetting, and sometimes dangerous, for family members.

The causes include:

- Personality changes rooted in mental changes. When someone with dementia becomes increasingly paranoid, frightened, or angry, he's more prone to explosive behavior.

- Loss of inhibition and social appropriateness. When angry impulses are tripped, self-control and self-censoring don't work the way they do in a healthy person.

- A situation that's frightening or threatening. This is related to brain changes. When he can't understand what the person helping him bathe is doing, for example (because he's lost the ability to recognize that he's dirty or what shower gel is) he may feel scared or violated. Any number of things can be misinterpreted. Being left alone for five minutes can feel like five hours when someone with dementia has lost the ability to track time, for example.

- A situation that makes your loved one feel insecure or uncomfortable. In addition to misperceptions, environmental realities can become upsetting — a noisy child, too much noise, an unfamiliar new aide.

- An underlying illness or physical problem. In some people, delirium can lead to aggressive behaviors. An infection, sleep deprivation, dehydration, or some other stressor can bring on delirium. In Carl's case, for example, the aggression was a new behavior that came on suddenly, rather than a pattern of behaviors over time — a red flag for a physical cause.

- An undetermined cause. Whatever the cause, he behaves in a rough, hostile, or even violent way: hitting, scratching, biting, pushing, slamming doors, throwing things, screaming, insulting, or resisting any attempt at assistance.

These behaviors are usually directed toward the hands-on helper but may also be done to others in the household, animals, or objects.

It's easy to misread the hostility and violence of someone with dementia as a lack of gratitude, rudeness, or meanness. Though those things may seem true on the surface, it's important to remember that the aggression is telling you something quite different. Lacking the ability to fully process what's happening or express feelings of discomfort well, these behaviors are a physical expression of mood: "I'm upset." "I'm angry." "I'm scared." "I'm so confused." "I feel overwhelmed and out of control."

TRY this:

In the moment:

- Hard as this can be, try not to take aggression personally and avoid reacting in kind. Raising your voice in response, threatening, or acting more forcefully can cause aggression to escalate. Your goal is the opposite: to reassure.

- Back off, rather than moving in to physically restrain. Not only might you get hurt if you try to subdue the person with dementia, but you'll cause him to fight harder. Backing off is defensive, protective — and, ultimately, gets the episode over faster.

- Stop doing whatever was happening at the moment. If you were trying to help him toilet or dress, withdraw. Give yourselves both a moment to calm down. If possible, don't return to that task at all for a while.

- Stick to a calm response and a pleasant expression. Even a smile — though that won't be your natural first response and may seem inappropriate — is helpful because body language is powerful and read better than your words. An angry response will be mirrored back.

- Also give a mild verbal response: "Everything's all right now." "Can I help you with something?" "I'm sorry you're upset." "Let's watch the birds out the window until you feel better."

- Step out of the room for a few minutes if you need a

moment to collect yourself. Better that objects are thrown or furniture is overturned than you risk injury yourself.

- When the outburst and its aftermath are over, avoid returning to the same activity. Try something pleasant or distracting — a root beer float, sitting on the porch, listening to some favorite music. Then try to repeat the fraught activity when he's in a calmer frame of mind. Try to avoid the exact thing you were doing at the time of the incident and do it in a slightly changed way (different tool, different approach, different order) to avoid an instant replay.

Tip: **"Figure out an arsenal of soothers that are things your person usually softens to. For us it's ice cream, singing, and a stuffed dog. Hard to be hostile when you're petting your favorite stuffed puppy." — R.E.**

To minimize further episodes:

- Look for changes in the home environment to see if you can identify what set off the aggression: Has a busy day left him tired? Is he sick or in pain? Is there a new helper who does things differently? Focus on what might be new or different. Beware of new medications. They can intensify aggression, either as a side effect or as an interaction with other meds. Take steps to avoid "trigger situations" once you've identified them.

- Reinforce routines and consistency. Everything you can do to create a secure, predictable environment can help. But know, too, that you can do everything right, and a confused mind may still imagine injustice or fear.

- Sometimes you can detect physical changes that indicate a blow-up is building. They vary by person, but clues might include a reddening face, a quavering or raised voice, and shaking hands. Stopping what you're doing (or changing the environment) and switching to something more calming can help avert an outburst.

120

- Report dangerous behaviors to his doctor. It's important to rule out underlying medical problems — not only delirium but also chronic pain or illnesses such as depression or other mental conditions that can be treated with medication.

Sometimes medications are used to control aggression, but be sure to weigh the benefits against the risks. Anti-anxiety medications and anti-depressants are used with aggression. So are anti-psychotics, although these raise the risk of stroke and death, and there's a strong shift away from their use for treating Alzheimer's patients. Every case should be assessed individually.

- Consider asking the doctor, a support group, the local Alzheimer's Association, or another outlet about training tips to deal with aggression and dementia (or difficult behaviors generally). Sometimes these presentations can teach you new ideas.

- Know that aggressive tendencies often worsen. If you ever don't feel safe, it may be time to consider out-of-home placement. Sadly, smaller spouses with a large mate who tends to lash out suddenly sometimes find this to be the case due to the sheer size disparity.

- Remove all firearms from the home. (Forty percent of veterans with dementia have them, reports the VA.) Even if your loved one has always used them wisely (or doesn't know how to use them because they belong to someone else), Alzheimer's changes everything. You can call your local sheriff's department to retrieve the gun for you. The Alzheimer's Association notes that they may want to see a statement of diagnosis from the person's doctor. If the person asks about a missing gun, you can try saying that a friend has "borrowed" it or it's been sent for a cleaning or repair. Alternately, you can have the gun made inoperable, but it's really safest to leave nothing to chance.

To help you cope:

- Don't be surprised when the person later acts (after a

hostile incident) as if nothing happened. He probably doesn't remember the outbursts. But if you persist in a grudging, angry mood — and it's a natural impulse to want to hold hostile acts against the perpetrator — he won't understand why and may parrot back your attitude. With dementia, he's not "acting innocent" afterward to manipulate you. That's why it's best to simply attribute the behavior to the disease and move on — provided, of course, that you safeguard yourself.

- Find outlets for your own feelings. You'll be upset. You'll want to react. That's only natural — and you should. It's just counterproductive for these reactions to be directed at the person with dementia. Far better to get your feelings out another way instead of lashing back or keeping them bottled up, where they can endanger your heart health and immune system. Punch pillows. Walk up and down stairs quickly. Have a friend or two on speed dial. Set up a secret dartboard in your bedroom. Write in a diary. But please, pick healthy outlets — turning to drugs or alcohol won't do you or the person with Alzheimer's much good in the long run.

- Know that it's common to feel you're living with a stranger, once aggression enters the picture — especially if he or she never showed such tendencies before. This can be a sad and isolating feeling, especially for spousal caregivers. Do reach out to a support group or online support network for the extra positive reinforcement you need.

o o o

Agitation and Meltdowns

Sarah often sits in a chair rocking, pulling yarn from a skein and loosely balling it, kneading it in her hands. Especially in the evening, this activity seems to soothe her. But at other times, she begins to rock harder and faster. Her hand motions grow wilder and she shouts random, often unintelligible, things.

Her grandchildren steer clear of Nana when she's like this. It's scary, they say.

WHY it happens:

Some people with dementia develop restlessness and mood swings. You may see nervous tics of repetitive actions or just a lot of twitchy, fidgety energy. Sometimes these behaviors simmer on low, other times they fester and build. Your loved one may seem to fly off the handle in a way that's out of proportion to the situation.

Sometimes agitation erupts into a catastrophic reaction — a fancy way of saying *meltdown*.

Agitation may also come out in the form of specific behaviors such as pacing, rummaging, cursing, screaming, and aggression. Agitation may also worsen late in the day (sundowning).

The main causes include:

- A psychiatric issue. Agitation is especially common when the person is paranoid, frightened, or angry. Less often, you see it in someone who's anxious or depressed. If you're seeing hallucinations and false beliefs, you may also see these agitated outbursts.

- A physical problem. When it's a new or sudden behavior, agitation can be a sign of delirium, which is caused by an underlying stressor to the body, such as infection or dehydration, or a reaction to a medication. This could be a new problem or a flare-up of a chronic disease. Disrupted sleep and pain can also lead to increased agitation.

- Stress from changes in the environment. Examples include a new caregiving aide, a disrupted routine, crowds or lots of visitors, too much noise, or a long wait at a busy doctor or dentist's office.

- A departure from routine or what's expected. Some people with dementia are highly anxious. A change in schedule (meals that are late) or a caregiver who's out of sight (in the basement doing laundry or off at work) can seem to set off a meltdown out of proportion to the incident itself.

- Being rushed or feeling pressured in any way.

- Boredom, lack of constructive activity, being left alone.

- Being hungry or tired can intensify a response to these stressors.

TRY this:

- When the agitation is a sudden, recent change, get a medical exam to rule out a physical cause.

- Don't respond in kind. It's critical to remain low-key to avoid revving up an agitated reaction further. Use a soothing, even voice to reassure: "You're all right. I'm right here. Nothing to worry about."

- Don't bother to scold or criticize someone who's behaving inappropriately. This isn't about what's "right." It's about getting back to calm.

- Avoid sudden movements. It can be a natural response to want to restrain or cordon off someone who's having a meltdown. But those actions can be perceived as a threat, adding a bellow's breath to the fire.

To avoid agitated responses:

- Arrange your lives around a routine. Predictability is reassuring and can ward off agitated responses.

- Do everything you can to keep daily life calm. In addition to routine, this means keeping noise levels down (including a blaring TV or radio) and keeping lights bright but soft (lower or close shades when sunlight creates glare).

- Avoid activities that cause undue frustration and challenge. You don't want to do everything for her, which can lead to boredom, but you do want to aim for a sweet spot where she can enjoy simple successes. Art projects can be an absorbing, calming way to pass time — as can listening to music, driving in a car, or making something (such as helping you make cookies) — so long as you keep the focus off the performance.

- Give yourself extra time for challenging activities, like going to the doctor. Feeling pressured or rushed can feed agitation.

o o o

Can't Make Decisions

Every Sunday, Jack took his grandfather to church and out to brunch. He liked spending time with Pappy and it was a way to give his parents, with whom Pappy lived, a needed break. "Why don't you find a table while I wash my hands?" he told the older man. They came here every week and usually sat by the windows. But when Jack exited the restroom, he was surprised to find Pappy still standing in the same spot.

He led him to their usual spot. "Look, they have both your favorites today, the maple waffles and the blueberry pancakes," Jack noted. When the waitress approached, Jack respectfully indicated his grandfather order first. "Well..." he said uncertainly. The waitress waited, pen poised. "Well let's see," said Pappy.

"Maple waffles? Blueberry pancakes?" Jack prompted helpfully. "Or do you feel like eggs today?"

"Well..."

Finally Jack ordered first. Then it was back to Pappy, who still frowned at the menu. "How about the waffles, you like those?" Jack finally suggested.

"Sure," said Pappy brightly. Waffles it was.

WHY it happens:

Decision-making involves remembering past preferences, weighing the pros and cons of the options, and assessing how you feel in the moment — mental calculations that a healthy brain can make instantly. But that seemingly simple ability to hold several ideas in mind at once and choose between them is a skill that dementia begins to erode even in the early stages of the disease.

For someone who has Alzheimer's, every decision, large or small — which table to choose in a restaurant, what to order, what to say or do next — can seem overwhelming, making the person feel frustrated and anxious.

The affected person may be afraid of making what will be seen as the "wrong" choice. Or he simply might not remember what the options are.

TRY this:

- Wait patiently for a reply rather than jumping in immediately. Feeling rushed can add to anxiety.

- If you see that someone is having trouble ,after a short spell, step in with a single suggestion or prompt: "Let's order the special." Or, "I'm having the tuna melt. You want one too?"

- Limit choices as much as possible to relieve unneeded stress. Especially eliminate open-ended choices. Avoid asking, "What do you want to eat?" or "What do you want to do today?" Better: "The special is spaghetti; shall we order that?" "Let's go to the park now."

- Know that when you give someone with Alzheimer's several choices, he may simply parrot back the last thing you said. So if you ask, "Do you want vanilla, strawberry, or chocolate ice cream?" the answer will likely be "chocolate." It can be helpful to offer up the last choice if you think it's what he prefers (or if that's what's easiest and makes no real difference).

- Simplify choices overall: Avoid buffets. Stock fewer clothes in the dresser and closet. Anticipate the person's preferences and find graceful ways to make choices for him, such as gifts or placing the best choices on top, where they'll be grabbed first.

o o o

Crying Jags (or Laughing Jags)

Millie's son can tell his mother is awake because the moaning cries rise up from her bed and crackle over the monitor to his room. She seems to wake up crying and often continues to moan, wail, and rock for hours. She pauses to eat or is sometimes distracted by the birds outside or her dog, but soon enough is wailing again.

WHY it happens:

There's often both an immediate reason for wailing and tears and a chronic one. Doctors call it "emotional lability" or emotional incontinence — an inability to manage emotional output. Less often, it's expressed as laughing jags.

In the immediate moment, the person feels a need to release emotion. The trigger can be anything, either specific (a perceived slight, a room that's too dark or too bright, too much noise) or, more often, broad (pain, boredom, loneliness, missing a deceased partner). For those who retain some awareness of their condition (or awareness that something's "not right" and life is a struggle), this knowledge alone can be enough to trigger tears.

One of two conditions usually underlies frequent crying:

1. Clinical depression. People with dementia are more prone than others to clinical depression, for reasons that aren't fully understood.

2. Pseudobulbar affect (PBA). This brain disorder can be caused by Alzheimer's or other kinds of brain injury, such as stroke or a head injury after a fall. The crying is not only socially inappropriate but often doesn't fit the circumstances (such as crying at a party). It's often mistaken for depression in someone with Alzheimer's. The National Stroke Association estimates that 1 million people may have PBA.

Crying jags aren't unusual in moderate or early severe stage dementia. Some people cry or laugh intermittently for hours at a stretch — an indicator of depression. With PBA, the bouts tend to be shorter (a matter of minutes) but can go on all day.

TRY this:

- Offer empathy: "You sound so sad. Can I help?" If you ask, "What's wrong?" the crying person will probably not be able to articulate her feelings.

- Provide physical support and affection — hugs, shoulder pats or rubs, and so on. Someone with dementia who's depressed has a deep need for both verbal and physical reassurance. Say, "It's okay. You're safe with me. Everything's all right."

- Mention the behavior to the doctor. It's important to look for other symptoms of depression, but also bring up the possibility of pseudobulbar affect, since it's under-diagnosed in Alzheimer's. Both PBA and clinical depression are treatable even in someone with moderate-stage Alzheimer's. Unfortunately both involve medication at a time in life when it's ideal to minimize medications, but depending on the severity of the behavior, treatment can make life more bearable for everyone.

Tip: **"We played a lot of slapstick old movies, like Charlie Chaplin, Abbott and Costello, Marx Brothers, and the Our Gang shows. When my mother was laughing, she didn't cry. It was like turning the spigot off for a while." — B.J.E.**

To help you cope:

- Know it's okay not to solve the problem. When a baby or small child cries, we're wired to rush in to fix it. But the crying jags of Alzheimer's can't always be fixed. Sometimes, you just have to endure them. Follow the steps above, and take solace that you've done all you can to be reassuring and to address the problem medically.

o o o

Follows You Everywhere (Shadowing)

When Stan gets up from his living room lounger to get some coffee, so does Stella, his wife of 51 years. "I'll bring it to you," he says.

"Okay," says Stella. But she follows him anyway. She follows him upstairs and downstairs, inside and outside. Lately, when he uses the bathroom, she's standing right outside the door waiting for him when he comes out.

WHY it happens:

A trusted family member can be a strong source of security and reassurance to someone with Alzheimer's — a kind of anchor in her increasingly confused world. You represent safety and steadfastness. You help her avoid embarrassment or frustration. In addition to the reassurance of your presence, she might be dependent on your knowledge and answers. Shadowing can increase if the person is bored.

For all these reasons, many people with dementia want to keep their primary caregiver in their direct line of vision at all times. They become almost your "shadow."

Some caregivers think shadowing happens because their loved one doesn't trust them, and it can certainly feel that way. But it's not about you. It's the disease feeding fear and anxiety about her disorienting experiences.

TRY this:

- Reinforce efforts to keep to a predictable household routine. Eating, resting, exercising, and leaving the house in the same order and at about the same times every day contribute to a feeling of security.

- See if you can identify a pattern: Does shadowing increase at a particular time of day? When certain people are around?

- Try saying something reassuring ("hello, dear"), rather

than showing annoyance or impatience. For stability's sake, it's important that you continue to be a calm social refuge.

- Make sure there are enough daily activities to absorb her. It's okay if they're repeats of things you just did yesterday or earlier in the day, like raking leaves or folding towels.

- Develop a handful of reassuring phrases: "It's a beautiful, calm day, Sweetheart." "You're safe and sound today." "You look wonderful today; I love you." Repetition of certain phrases works well for many.

- Use music to soothe. Try preparing a calming or reassuring playlist that the person can sit and listen to through headphones (Headphones aren't necessary, but they can be handy if you get tired of listening to certain tracks over and over.)

- Try not to go out of sight for long periods of time. People with dementia can't track time well. Five minutes might seem like an hour. If you must be out of the room for a while (such as to shower or to do laundry in a basement), check in verbally every few minutes.

- Try setting a timer when you take a shower or have a similar task: "When the timer goes off, I'll be done." Use a timer that makes a reassuring ticking sound and place it where the person can watch it. When you return, say, "See, I came back just like I said I would when the timer dinged."

Tip: "I used a baby monitor when I had to leave the room. I would keep talking into it so my mom could hear my voice — I'd tell her where I was and that I'd be right back." — J.G.

To help you cope:

- Be sure to arrange respite for yourself every other day or so — even if only for an hour or two while you go for a walk or have a cup of coffee with a friend. Don't think that because your loved one is so dependent on you that your constant presence is an absolute necessity. She'll manage well enough under someone else's temporary attentive care

- Know that even when you love the person with dementia dearly, even when you've spent a lifetime together, shadowing is different. Being shadowed can become claustrophobic and stressful; humans need some privacy! Being able to have someone else spend short amounts of time with the affected person is critical for your mental health.

o o o

Hallucinates (Sees and Hears Things That Aren't There)

"Good morning," I said as I entered the kitchen.

My mother-in-law, in her mid-80s, smiled. "Did you see that grizzly bear in the yard?"

"No, where?" I asked in surprise and mild panic, looking out the kitchen window into her suburban New Jersey backyard.

"Last night! It was standing up, right over there! I called the police!"

"Last night?" I asked, confused. "Police?" She had gone to bed first, and it had been a peaceful evening.

"Oh yes! A bunch of men came over with guns!"

As it happened, there was no police report of any such incident, no word of bears in the neighborhood — and, in fact, no bear. — P.S.S.

WHY it happens:

Hallucinations — seeing, hearing, feeling, smelling, or even tasting things that aren't there — usually occur in the later stages of dementia due to brain changes and difficulty telling fantasy from reality. A person may hear voices and even chat or argue with a long-dead relative. Another may feel like her hair is on fire or smell fire where there is none. Still another person might claim to see ants in her food. Any of these things seem absolutely real to the person with dementia. They may or may not be upsetting.

These perception changes can worsen in the evening. Triggers can include stress, unusual noise or light, or lack of sleep. Hearing or vision problems can intensify the misperception.

Hallucinations can also be a feature sign of delirium, especially if they're sudden in onset. (These delirium hallucinations are caused by an underlying stressor, such as an infection or pain.) Some medications can also cause false perceptions.

Estimates range widely as to how common hallucinations are in Alzheimer's; studies report anywhere from 10 to 60 percent of patients have some kind at some point. (Hallucinations are even more common in another type of dementia, Lewy Body.) And people with Alzheimer's who experience hallucinations are at increased risk for faster cognitive and functional decline, studies show.

TRY this:

- Consider other physical changes that might be related and get a medical check-up to rule out possible causes apart from dementia, such as a urinary tract infection, a bad medication reaction, or dehydration.

- Assess the impact of the hallucination. You don't have to do much if it's not upsetting the person (not causing fear or agitation, for example) or leading to dangerous behavior (such as refusing to eat or leading her outdoors where she's prone to wandering off).

- Avoid correcting her or trying to prove the illogic of the perception. Realize that it seems quite real to her and that she can't be argued out of it.

- See if you can make a connection to reality that might be triggering the hallucination. For example, a shadow of moving branches might be perceived as an intruder. Sounds of a violent TV show might be mistaken for events happening in the room. The hum of an air conditioner may sound like voices. There isn't always a logical connection, but it's worth considering in case you can fix the problem easily — for example by turning on a light or turning off the TV.

- Acknowledge the imaginary perception. Comment in away that's matter of fact and reassuring. A little white lie of agreement is okay here ("I'm glad to hear the police took care of it and everything is safe and back to normal. Do you want toast for breakfast?")

- Use empathetic phrasing that plays back the person's feelings: "That must have been scary." "I can see that you're not happy about that."

- If the hallucination is upsetting, assure that you'll take care of it. Remind her with words and a soothing hug that she's safe with you.

- Go along with what you reasonably can. One woman put out leftovers for imaginary cats; her daughter emptied the dishes when her mom napped. Another caregiver provided a flashlight for her dad to chase the "little people under my bed."

- Distract with a pleasant experience, such as a favorite snack or a game of cards. Play soothing music or introduce a change of scenery by moving to a different room or going outside.

- Avoid reminding the person of the incident later or bring it up again. Often the person hallucinated quickly forgets even a startling experience. (The rest of the household might be shaken up for awhile!)

- If hallucinations become disruptive and constant, such as interfering with sleep, consult the doctor. Anti-psychotic medications may help, but because they're powerful drugs, they're always considered a last, not first, line of defense.

To help you cope:

- Remember that many hallucinations are harmless, so always start by asking yourself: Is the problem here how the perception is affecting my relative, such as disrupting sleep? Or is it that she's doing or saying things that (embarrassingly, to you) make her seem a little cuckoo?

o o o

Has Delusions (False Accusations and Ideas)

"You hussy!" Leonard hissed at Lou, his wife of 53 years, when she entered the room.

"What did you call me?" she said, taken aback.

"I saw you, sneaking off with that gardener! I was watching you through the window! You didn't think I saw you, but I know all about your flirting and your running around!"

Gardener? Running around? Lou had never so much as looked at another man before. And they'd never had a gardener at their tiny suburban bungalow. "Stop talking nonsense!" she admonished. But Leonard only sneered at her more, until she burst into tears and had to leave the room.

Stepping onto the front porch for air, she realized that shortly before the tirade, she'd gone to the front yard to give the boy across the street some lemonade and some money. His mother had asked him to start cutting their lawn after noticing it getting shaggy. Leonard couldn't do it any more and Lou seldom had time herself. She'd been so grateful — how could Leonard think she was flirting with the kid? He was all of 13!

WHY it happens:

Because someone with dementia has lost the ability to reason and make accurate judgments, he may blame others for any confusion or difficulty he encounters. Things he can't make sense of leave him feeling anxious. Can't find his glasses? *That aide stole them!* Doesn't recognize a neighbor who's mowing his lawn for him? *He must be the fella sneaking around with my wife!*

Known as *paranoid delusions*, false accusations can take many forms. Among the most common irrational beliefs for people with Alzheimer's: accusing someone of stealing, accusing a spouse of adultery, believing the house is being invaded, claiming that family members have been replaced by impostors. Nearly one in three people with Alzheimer's have delusions.

Delusions can happen at any stage of Alzheimer's but have been found to be most common in the moderate stage of disease, as the ability to distinguish reality erodes.

TRY this:

- Skip trying to prove your innocence or berate the person for making an outrageous claim. The more you protest, the more fixed this belief often becomes.

- Let the person talk. Listen attentively and empathetically.

- Ask questions that encourage details: "What did she do?" "Where did they go?" "When did you notice your money was missing?" (Avoid the one you're itching to ask most, though. You won't get any kind of useful answer to "Why?") You're not doing this to collect evidence to "solve" the mystery. Rather, you're validating the person's perception — stepping into his world — by letting him share his thoughts, and you might get insight into the origin of the belief. For example, he might tell you he knew when his wife was replaced by an alien because her hair is different (and you know she just got a haircut).

- Avoid agreeing to a falsehood. This is a situation where an agreeable white lie rarely pays off. You might make things worse ("You think she was stealing, too? I'm going to fire her right now!"). More likely, the person with dementia can't process what you're saying or may quickly forget and start the loop of accusing again.

- Rely on humor: "Sorry, you're stuck with me, dear — you know I've always been a one-man gal." Or, "I don't know why, but Mom insists you're mates for life."

- Provide a simple solution, if you can: "Here are your glasses." If certain objects go "missing" often, consider getting multiples of them.

- Give lots of reassurance (without disputing the delusion): "It's safe now." "I love you." "We found your missing ring."

- Keep a few dollars or an inactive credit card in the wallet of someone who often accuses others of stealing. Often families remove these items for safety's sake, but that can have the unintended effect of upsetting the person, who fears he's been robbed because he's used to seeing money and cards in a wallet.

- Distract. Change the subject or move to another room. "Let's talk about this some more after we check the bird feeder." "Before we look for the missing candlesticks, let's get something to eat for energy."

- Assure the accused, if someone other than you, that this is the disease talking. Reassure him or her that you value their presence and don't believe the falsity.

To help you cope:

- Separate your feelings from the accusation. Realize that these delusions have almost nothing to do with the quality of the relationship between the accuser and the accused. A beloved grandson might be accused of stealing money. The spouse in a long-happy marriage, who is a devoted caregiver, might get pegged as an adulterer.

o o o

Hoarding, Hiding, and Clutter

Joanne's mother, Doris, had always been a bit disorganized and messy. Over the years, piles of papers seemed to grow on her desk, atop the kitchen counter, on the floor around her favorite lounge chair. At first, Joanne and her sister Beth just wrote the habit off as messiness. They got used to hearing Doris say, "I'm saving that to look at later," or "You never know when you might need it."

Eventually Doris began showing other symptoms of dementia, from forgetfulness to critical financial mistakes. Meanwhile the clutter grew. Doris began to save empty yogurt containers that she'd clean and stack on the windowsill. When her daughters asked why she was doing it, she'd brush them off: "Stay out of my kitchen!"

Doris, who was divorced, still lived alone. One day Beth visited and found empty yogurt containers — not all of them clean — on the windowsills of the dining room. She used the bathroom, and more yogurt cups lined the sill there. The house seemed full of more yogurts than her mother could have possibly eaten. Coming out of the bathroom with an armful to throw away, Doris had a fit. "Stop! Stop!" she cried, yanking her daughter's arm so the cups fell to the floor.

"Mom! These are dirty!" Beth explained. Doris hit her.

Beth retreated to her car and whipped out her cellphone. "Joanne," she said to her sister. "We've got to talk!"

WHY it happens:

Starting very early in the disease, people sometimes acquire multiples of certain types of objects to an unusual degree, beyond ordinary collecting. They may simply forget they've bought a certain kind of salad dressing, for example, and buy it every time they shop until suddenly there are a dozen identical bottles in the cupboard.

As judgment erodes, they may be reluctant to throw anything away — not only necessities, but things that are no longer needed, even trash. Junk mail, empty tissue boxes, clothes, and other objects pile up.

They may hide objects — often in unusual or illogical places — to keep them safe. Conversely, some people keep things out where they're visible (toiletries on tabletops, clothes draped over stair railings) in order to keep them safe and not lose them.

About one in five people with Alzheimer's are thought to be true hoarders — those who obsessively collect and save objects to an extent that's potentially dangerous.

Unlike objects in a conventional collector's collection, these things may have no value (sentimental, monetary, or otherwise) and the practice can take over the person's life to a degree that's socially isolating or physically dangerous, such as clutter that represents a fire or tripping hazard.

Sometimes the objects are confined to one space. Sometimes there's clutter everywhere. Or objects might be hidden in unusual spots.

Common things people with Alzheimer's hoard, according to a study in the *American Journal of Geriatric Psychiatry*, include papers, daily necessities (such as toiletries), newspapers and magazines, plastic bags, broken umbrellas, old clothes, food, and garbage.

Causes of hoarding include:

- An obsessive-compulsive disorder that may have existed separately from the dementia. (People who were prone to clutter before dementia tend to get worse.)

- Cognitive changes. She can no longer distinguish between what's worth saving and what isn't, and can't make decisions. Memory loss may lead to a habit of misplacing objects and forgetting where they're stored.

- Boredom or lack of healthier stimulation

- Anxiety. Fearing loss (or expressing loss), the person gets security from setting aside random objects. Hoarding is related to rummaging, as the person later searches for the objects and the mere act of touching them provides security.

TRY this:

- When the person is asleep, thin the collection. Leave several items, so it doesn't feel completely decimated, yet is safer and more manageable. Getting rid of everything at once can be distressing and counterproductive. Throw away food items that aren't safe to save. Whatever you throw away should be removed from the home completely — not placed in the garbage or even the trashcan at the end of the driveway, where it can be searched for and retrieved.

- Repeat clean-ups regularly. Without ongoing help, the clutter will quickly return.

- If asked where items have gone, offer an explanation that the hoarder may respond to positively: You donated them to a family in need, you gave them to a niece for a birthday gift, her church asked for donations.

- Don't bother providing additional space or equipment for organizing the clutter (extra tables, baskets, bins, etc.). The problem is that the person can no longer organize. Extra space will only result in extra clutter.

- Check preferred hiding spots regularly. Many people develop certain quirky "go to" spots to hide things: kitchen canisters (for trash, rather than sugar and flour), certain drawers, under mattresses, laundry hampers, underused closets, in the bushes outside.

- If you see her rummaging around, suggest these go-to hiding places. Even these favorite spots may be forgotten!

- Plug up the sources of the incoming stuff, if you can. For example, cancel newspaper or magazine subscriptions, block home shopping channels, close problematic credit card accounts.

o o o

Phones Over and Over

"It's Mom. When are you coming over?"

"Mom, I came by this morning. I'm at work now."

"Oh....sure...are you coming by later? I need you to look at my toaster."

"Yes, Mom, you already called me twice about that."

Tony's mother, Flora, lives alone ten minutes from his house. Even though he stops by before and after work, she's begun to call him increasingly often during the day and in the evening.

"It's Mom. Turn on channel 20. It's the funniest thing!"

"I can't, Mom, I'm at work."

"Oh, okay. Then why did you call me?"

WHY it happens:

The telephone is a kind of umbilical cord for many people with Alzheimer's, representing security — pick it up, and there you are. When feeling insecure, lonely, scared, or simply when thinking of you, the person places a call. Worsening memory makes her unable to remember that she called earlier (once, twice, a dozen times).

Familiar, long-dialed numbers — yours, the doctor's office, a friend's — tend to be called most often. A single-button speed-dial system makes it especially easy to call those individuals.

Some people dial 911 repeatedly to get a live human to talk to (not about an emergency), maybe because "911" is a deeply ingrained number.

Or calling becomes a behavioral tic, a form of repetitive behavior.

Other common phone problems:

- *She can't find and pick up the phone.*

- WHY: A modern telephone might be confused for a TV remote or other gadget. Impaired thinking makes her unable to connect the ring with the need to pick it up. Or she may pick it up but not press the right button to activate a call.

- *She answers the phone but doesn't speak.*

- WHY: She doesn't recognize the disembodied voice. Or she has bad hearing on top of the dementia, and can't hear it.

- *She answers the phone but doesn't take a message.*

- WHY: She may think she'll remember (but never does). Or she lacks the wherewithal to get a pen and go through the motions of writing down what's said.

TRY this:

The right solution depends on your specific situation, but these ideas may help:

- Switch to a phone with number recognition display (caller ID) or set a specific ring tone for your relative, so you can decide which calls to answer. Especially at night, let the message go to voicemail and decide whether it's a crisis or not. Your loved one may grow frustrated by not hearing your actual voice and begin to call less (although others will call even more often).

- Cancel the landline and use your cellphone only if you live in the same house. That way, your loved one can't call out if she's a repetitive caller.

- Claim you're making the switch to "save money" — an appeal that works for many Depression-era children.

- Place phones only in the rooms where the person with Alzheimer's doesn't go, such as your bedroom and the basement.

- Use call forwarding to send home calls to your cellphone.

- Turn down ringers. This may prevent the phone from being answered but not prevent outgoing calls — though hearing less ringing may make the phone less top-of-mind for the person with dementia.

- For people with early-stage disease, look into easy-to-use models that have visual cue buttons to easily identify family members or emergency help.

- Another option, for those who call often: dial-less phones that receive calls but don't permit calling out.

- Be aware that not being able to use the phone properly — whether from overuse or avoidance — is a sign that someone who lives alone can't dial emergency services or 911 as needed, a red flag for being unable to live independently.

To help you cope:

- You might feel guilty about not answering every call, but remember that you have a life to lead, especially at work and at night.

o o o

Paces, Shows Signs of Restlessness

You can tell where Kara's mother, Katrina, likes to walk. The carpet is noticeably dirtier in a distinct path from her bedroom, down the hall to the den, around the perimeter of the den, and back to her bedroom. Around 3 o'clock every afternoon, Katrina rises from the sofa and begins to walk this pattern as intently as if she were prayer-walking in a labyrinth.

"She does it for an hour or longer — I guess until she's tired," says Kara. "She used to welcome my kids, her grandkids, home from school, and they'd have a snack in the den. I wonder if that's what she's thinking about. But if you ask her, she ignores you. It's as if she isn't even aware of what she's doing."

WHY it happens:

Pacing — walking aimlessly or in a particular pattern around the home — is a common repetitive behavior or *perseveration* (the term for this behavior). Other examples include rocking, making repeated phone calls, picking at skin, and rummaging.

Pacing is typically caused by:

- Anxiety or another form of distress. What's bothering the person may be recent (a new caregiver, noise) or some long unresolved issue from the past.

- Boredom, feeling unproductive. Someone once used to a busy life may pace.

- A need to use the bathroom — but an inability to say so.

- A habitual impulse to move. Former exercise-walkers, runners, or swimmers, for example, may pace if they can no longer walk outside for safety or stamina reasons.

- A cognitive glitch that may or may not be related to the above; the person "gets stuck" on a particular behavior pattern.

TRY this:

- First address possible immediate needs: Lead the person to the toilet and see if she needs to go, for example.

- Reinforce comforting routines, and make sure physical activity is included.

- Ignore pacing that seems to calm, rather than agitate, someone with Alzheimer's. But look for alternate activities to counter possible boredom.

- Make the house safer for walking. If you haven't already done so, remove throw rugs, arrange furniture to make clear pathways, and get rid of clutter and low-to-the-ground hazards such as magazine racks, plants, and extension cords.

- Install night lighting. Illuminate preferred safe paths — especially the hallways and rooms most used — with motion-sensitive nightlights, for example.

O O O

Picks at Skin, Clothes, or Small Objects

Ryan began to feel embarrassed about taking his father out in public — the older man's arms were dotted with red sores and half-healed scabs. He'd developed the habit of scratching at a dry spot on his skin while watching TV in the evening. Then when blood appeared, he'd pick at the edges. After a scab began to form, he'd pick at that, too, so old sores never completely healed even as he continued creating new ones.

When Ryan applied bandages, his dad picked those off, too.

WHY it happens:

Picking can refer to obsessively handling any number of different things: skin, labels, lint, pilling on sweaters, sticks, peeling paint. Some people pick at their hair or scalp.

Someone who picks constantly might feel anxious about something in his current life, or something deep in his past. Either way, the repetitive activity is soothing. He may not seem aware of the habit. For some chronic pickers, the compulsion is a way of gaining a sense of control in a life where they may feel little control (not unlike teenagers who cut themselves or those with an eating disorder, like bulimia).

Often, scratching the skin is triggered because of an irritant or a skin condition that makes skin dry and uncomfortable. Older skin can already be dry and fragile. Becoming dehydrated can also affect skin. In those situations, it's not unusual for someone with Alzheimer's to scratch or pick until skin bleeds.

TRY this:

- Mention skin-picking to the doctor, who can rule out or treat dry skin caused by a medication or other reversible cause.

- Is it a new behavior? Consider whether a new bath product, laundry detergent or dryer sheet, cold weather, or medication might be irritating skin. Bed bugs, lice, or mosquito bites can also cause itching.

- Be sure a chronic picker cleans his hands often, to prevent infection, and keep nails trimmed short. Apply a topical antibiotic such as Neosporin to open sores and try to cover with a bandage. Re-check often, as it also might get picked off.

- Apply lots of moisturizers designed for dry skin to keep skin soft, especially after bathing. Be sure he drinks enough to ward off dehydration's drying effects.

- Help him dress in long-sleeve shirts to cover skin. Lightweight cotton is most comfortable. A wool, cashmere, or synthetic sweater that pills can be a safer substitute to pick at than skin. Someone who picks at the scalp may consent to wearing a hat and lose the habit if the hands are diverted. For an entrenched habit, try clothing that fastens in the back and can't be removed.

- Offer alternatives to keep the hands busy. Examples: finger puppets, worry beads, rubber de-stressing balls, a rubber-band ball, yarn to wind or a simple crocheting project, a toolbox to organize, clothes or towels to fold, lotion or nail polish to apply, something textured to hold that can't be picked (such as a textured rubber ball), a gadget to use (like an iPod), a junk drawer to organize.

- For more advanced-stage disease, consider an activity apron or lap pillow — a coverall apron or pillow designed for tactile stimulation, with different textures and things to handle sewn right on the fabric. Try searching online for "Alzheimer's activity apron."

- Reinforce a sense of meaning and purpose. Find ways to involve the person in household activities and express your gratitude for his efforts often.

- Try to remind yourself that except for picking at skin or nails, which is dangerous because it can lead to infection, the habit is harmless.

o o o

Rummages

"What are you looking for, Ma?" asks Kate.

"Oh, I'll find it soon," Kate's mother, Dorothy, says evasively as she goes on opening and closing drawers, riffling through papers, old makeup, pencils, balls of string, and a jumble of other unrelated objects. The rummaging tends to start in the evening and can go on for an hour or more. Eventually, Dorothy picks out something — an old sock, masking tape, a turkey baster — and announces, "Ah, just what I was looking for!"

Some nights, though, she never "finds" the thing she thinks she needs.

WHY it happens:

Rummaging — restlessly and repeatedly going through drawers, papers, toolboxes, or similar collections of materials — is one of many different repetitive behaviors some people with dementia show.

It can have several different (sometimes overlapping) causes:

- Agitation or anxiety. Moving the hands around is a way to channel a lack of ease.

- Boredom. It's simply something to do.

- Lack of exercise. Not moving around enough can come out as restless behaviors.

- Feeling vulnerable, upset, or otherwise nervous. As with other continuous behaviors, rummaging can be calming.

- Chronic hoarding. Someone who's a hoarder may be searching for a "saved" object.

TRY this:

- Look for a trigger. Does the behavior begin or increase when your loved one is tired or in the company of new people? Is there too much background noise? Could it be related to being left alone or not having anything to do?

- Try not to dwell on the behavior. Avoid saying, "Don't do that!" or "What on earth are you looking for?" Instead focus on the person more generally, her mood, and the circumstances of his day.

- Ask if she's looking for something. It's possible that she has an item in mind but has forgotten where it is (or even what the object is). You don't need to go along with it to the point where you're rummaging, too. But a kind normal response can be reassuring.

- Suggest that a chronic hoarder look in her favorite "go to" hiding places. Common sites include a hamper or laundry bag, special drawers, or unusual spots like sugar bowls and kitchen canisters.

- When in doubt, take the behavior as a sign that your loved one needs comfort and reassurance. Offer a hug.

- Accept rummaging that isn't disruptive as a curious function of the disease and let the person have at it. Just be sure to remove anything dangerous that could be handled and misused, such as sharp knives or guns.

- Redirect problematic rummaging (such as messing up critical work papers or rummaging in garbage) to a better alternative. Try creating a dedicated box or junk drawer of similar materials, or introduce something else the person may enjoy handling. Things that have worked for some caregivers include coins, buttons, office miscellany, papers or junk mail, kitchen utensils, and mixed beans to sort. Be sure the person doesn't put the objects in her mouth; if that's a problem, choose accordingly.

- Find other ways to channel nervous energy that involve the hands: balling yarn, working with hand tools, playing with worry beads or knotted string, filling or putting stamps on envelopes, peeling potatoes or carrots.

o o o

Sundowning (Worsening Behaviors in the Evening)

Len has come to dread dinnertime. He likes to eat well enough — it's what starts happening as he prepares the meal, and what comes after, that's getting harder to take. His wife, Doris, starts saying the craziest things.

"Watch out for the creepies!" she often says to herself or to him (he isn't sure which). "The creepies are coming! I know it, I know it!" She can't articulate who, or what, "creepies" are. She doesn't talk about them during the day — if he asks, she looks at him like he's crazy.

He used to turn on the TV so she could watch while he cooked, but she began to see the creepies in news programs and laundry commercials. Now he has her sit in the kitchen with him, but she can't sit still — she peeks out the windows and peers into cupboards. By day, Len can have a back-and-forth conversation with Doris. But not at dinnertime or after. For the rest of the evening, until she finally falls asleep exhausted, well past 10 (and well past when Len is worn out), she'll be wringing her hands and talking nonsense.

WHY it happens:

The name for an onset of increased agitation, confusion, and/or aggression in late afternoon or evening — also called "sundown syndrome" and "sundowner's" — comes from the time of day it tends to strike, typically late afternoon, after the sun goes down. Someone with dementia who sundowns may pace, wander, lash out, yell, show mood swings, hallucinate, show increased paranoia, or become unusually resistant. (These behaviors can also happen separately from sundowning at any time of day.)

Researchers aren't entirely sure what triggers sundown syndrome but think it's related to a disruption of the internal body clock. All our bodies follow circadian rhythms, which govern when we sleep and awaken, our activity, and the hormonal reactions that help our bodies run properly. For unknown reasons, people with dementia have a disturbed body clock. There's some research to show that aging eyes (even in people without dementia) take in less sunlight, which may affect circadian rhythms.

Researchers point to these other possible causes or triggers for sundowning:

- A drop in blood pressure

- Hunger or a change in glucose levels

- Reduced sleep needs (or, conversely, being overtired)

- Pain

- Poor hearing or vision, which alters perception

- Depression.

Several of these factors are probably connected, researchers think. For example, someone with dementia and macular degeneration (an eye condition) may become more confused and upset by evening shadows, especially if tired.

Sundowning happens more often in fall and winter (when there's less daylight) and as dementia progresses.

TRY this:

- Try to identify patterns other than time of day. Does the setting sun hit mirrors or windows in a bothersome way, for example? Does the house get noisier at dinnertime as family members come home?

- If you can identify a trigger, work to eliminate it. Take the person to a quiet room when the kids come home, for example. Trim back bushes or branches that create eerie shadows.

- Expose your loved one to ample sunlight, especially early in the day. Make sure she gets strong morning sun, either by going outside or sitting near a window with the curtains open. On cloudy days, try placing a full-spectrum fluorescent lamp (2,500 to 5,000 lux) a few feet away for two or three hours in the morning, say, while she's watching TV.

- Gentle exercise or an outing in the morning or midday may help her feel more tired at the end of the day, especially if you curb long naps.

- Try not to let her fall into a sleep-wake schedule that's wildly out-of-synch with yours. Waken her relatively early in the day, even if it would be more convenient to let her sleep. Minimize all-afternoon napping.

- Reinforce routines. If things happen at a different time every day, the sundowning might worsen.

- If dinner will be served late, make sure to serve a sustaining snack, such as a complex carbohydrate or protein (like 100 percent whole-wheat toast with almond butter or some string cheese and crackers).

- As evening nears, increase soothing sleep cues. Play soft music instead of TV (news shows and reality shows can be especially jarring). Serve warm milk or cocoa, or ice cream. Draw the shades and turn off some indoor lighting. Offer a hand massage while you have a quiet talk or listen to music.

- Secure the exits with motion sensors, locks, or gates to prevent nighttime wandering out of the house.

- Make sure eyeglasses and hearing aids are clean and functioning (someone with dementia will probably neglect to do this) and that the prescriptions are current. An eye exam could reveal an undiagnosed problem, such as macular degeneration, for example.

- If aggression or other behaviors become hard to handle, mention sundowning to the affected person's doctor. Mood stabilizers or the hormone melatonin may be effective. Beware of using over-the-counter sleep aids, however; these can interact badly with Alzheimer's medications. Best: Take all medications to the doctor so that they can be reviewed individually and together. Some might not be necessary.

To help you cope:

• Reassure yourself that you're not crazy (or faint of heart) if sundowning is a big problem for you. Depending on how it plays out in a given person, it can be extremely taxing to deal with and disrupt the sleep of the entire household. In extreme cases, it can be the "straw that breaks the camel's back," making home care impossible. Try as many behavioral interventions as you can, then consider medication. At the very least, persistent disruptive sundowning is a red flag to access more help or begin to consider what you'll do when you can no longer provide care at home.

o o o

Trouble Using Familiar Gadgets

My Dad was a veritable Mr. Gadget. A mechanical engineer and a gifted car mechanic, he was a natural and enthusiastic early adopter of color TVs, portable TVs, pocket calculators, CD players, car phones, cell phones, camcorders, and more types of tools and automotive gadgets than a low-techie like me could possibly identify. Into his 80s, he embraced desktop computers, digital cameras, home photo printers, and iPods.

It was especially distressing, then, to watch him at the bank one day deep into his dementia: He repeatedly jammed the wrong plastic card into an ATM. Finally, with help, he inserted the correct bank card — only to be baffled by the buttons and options that followed.

Another time, a stopped clock drove him crazy. He checked his watch often and knew its time was wrong. And his instinct to tinker and repair remained strong. So he kept taking the clock off the wall to "fix" it. But by the time he pried off the back cover and inspected it, he could go no farther. He'd grunt and touch the control knob but utterly lacked the wherewithal to actually replace the batteries, re-set the time, replace the back, and return the clock to the wall. Over and over, I'd find the abandoned repair job, put it back together, and replace it on the wall. (In retrospect....I know! Why didn't I just get it repaired or hide it from view?!)

The telephone was an ongoing source of stress. When my mom would motion for him to pick up an extension, he'd invariably choose one of several different TV and stereo remotes and start talking into it. (Well, they were all black and long and full of buttons.) — P.S.S.

WHY it happens:

Understanding of many common objects recedes as Alzheimer's progresses. The mastery of gadgetry we take for granted — phones, laptops, VCRs, microwaves — often come first. In part it's because these are relatively complex tools that require an ability to follow a sequence of steps to use and a memory of the details involved, such as what a particular button represents. Obviously this is a more notable symptom in someone who was versed in these gadgets before; some people were never adept at them. It's important to focus on what has *changed*.

People with Alzheimer's lose the ability to sequence their actions. Eventually, they stop recognizing objects for what they are — even simple tools, such as a toothbrush, can confuse them.

TRY this:

- Be patient if you get a new version of an old device (such as a new remote with different buttons). Learning new things is very difficult by mild stage dementia. Even someone well versed in gadgets may find it difficult to learn how to use a device that's slightly different.

- Try using memory aids: Circle the "on" button with permanent marker; leave a note boiled down to two simple instructions ("Press red button. Then press yellow one."). Over time, even these may be hard to follow.

- Avoid storing similar gadgets near each other. A cell phone and a camera, or a house phone and a TV remote, for example, are often confused for each other.

- Look for simplified versions of devices. There are laptops that only do e-mail, "memory" phones whose buttons have pictures of the people most often dialed, and dial-less telephones that can be answered but not dialed. Learning to use even simple new devices can be challenging, however.

- Try not to criticize mistakes. Just gently offer your help: "Let me see if I can do it."

- Phase out the use of gadgets that create consternation and confusion.

Tip: **"To give my mom something to look at without her having to change channels, I put on long, two- to three-hour DVDs. Sometimes nature shows, sometimes cartoons. No commercials and no buttons to push." — J.M.L.**

o o o

Undresses in Public

"I'm hot," Mildred announced to her family, gathered for her birthday. Ten minutes later, she reappeared in the dining room. She'd changed from her heavy sweater into a light blouse — and nothing else. No pants, no panties.

Her daughter Marie shrieked. Her grandchildren started snickering. "What's the matter? Haven't you ever felt like being free?" Mildred said, waggling her wrinkled hips.

Says Marie: "Not a week later, Mom said she was hot at a restaurant and started to undo the snaps on her blouse, right at the table. She got the whole thing off almost before any of us realized it. When the poor waiter, a teenage boy, stared, she said, 'Haven't you ever seen a bra before, honey?'"

WHY it happens:

The checks-and-balances in the brain that prevent her from doing or saying whatever she feels like in the moment erode as part of the brain changes brought on by dementia. She may gradually lose the ability to recognize what's socially appropriate behavior along with the ability to stop herself. This loss of inhibitions is known as *disinhibition.*

She may start to disrobe because she:

- Feels too hot

- Is uncomfortable (itchy tag, bra too snug, scratchy fabric, etc.)

- Needs to use the bathroom

- Is sexually aroused

- Is bored.

TRY this:

- See if you can connect the behavior to a specific cause you can remedy, such as scratchy fabrics or the temperature in the room.

- Be low-key and matter-of-fact: "No, we don't do that here. Let me help you find a shirt that's cooler (or that you like better)." If you're in public or with others, cover the person and calmly and quietly escort her to a more private place. Some caregivers travel with a shawl for handy coverage in a pinch.

- Use redirection to give her something else to do. You may be able to persuade someone with advanced dementia to wear a "busy apron" onto which zippers, buttons, ribbons, dangling keys, and other hand-occupying things have been sewn.

- Know that clothing can irritate older, dry skin, so the person wants to shed it. Look for soft, seamless undergarments, sweatpants, and tops. All cotton is usually more comfortable than synthetic. Cashmere and fleece are softer and less itchy than wool.

- If it's becoming a chronic problem, try coveralls, jumpsuits, or shirts without buttons or that button in the back.

- Search online for "Alzheimer's clothing." Some makers offer special clothes that are designed to be hard to get out of. Beware, though, that these choices can be counterproductive if the person needs to use the bathroom often.

- Ask the doctor to review medications that may be contributing to dry skin or for suggestions for ultra-rich moisturizers.

To help you cope:

- Let go of worries about propriety and what others might think. Your loved one isn't trying to embarrass you or mortify you. When you remember it's just the disease at work, it's easier to find the calm you'll need to handle it.

o o o

Upset by Reflection in Mirror

Lately Jack had become reluctant to take a shower. "I don't like being watched," he complained. His wife, Ann, assured him that she wasn't watching; she would just be waiting outside the door like always, with a warm towel and fresh pajamas. "I'm being stalked. I know it," he insisted.

One day as Jack and Ann walked down the hall, he grabbed her arm and froze. "Don't move! There he is again! Call the police!" Ann panicked and tried to follow his gaze. A framed mirror hung in an alcove at the end of the hall. Her heart sank. The "intruder" Jack saw — as well as, she then realized, the "bathroom stalker" — was her husband's own reflection.

WHY it happens:

Just as someone loses the ability to recognize longtime acquaintances, he can lose the ability to register his own reflection as himself. A moving image in a mirror may not register as a reflection of someone he knows in the house but instead seem like a stranger.

Some people befriend "the person in the mirror." They have pleasant conversations with their reflection. If it's a source of entertainment and pleasure and doesn't cause him to grow agitated or upset, there's no reason to discourage the behavior.

One caregiver reported finding her mother washing her face — only it was the face of her reflection!

TRY this:

- Remove or cover (with a large towel, cloth, or curtain) any mirrors that have become bothersome.

- If a medicine cabinet has a mirrored door, try replacing it with a solid door or removing it and leave the open shelving. Remove any dangerous substances, such as medications the person with dementia might take accidentally.

- If it's a large wall-sized mirror (as in many modern bathrooms), try hanging a curtain or shower curtain rod over the top, so the curtain can be open or closed. It may seem very odd to you or your guests, but to your loved one, the mirror may come to be "out of sight, out of mind."

- Switch to using hand mirrors or portable makeup mirrors for yourself. Store a full-length mirror inside a closet, where it can't be accidentally glimpsed.

- Look to see if reflective glass on a painting or framed poster is having the same effect. You might need to relocate the piece.

- If someone continues to talk about people "watching" or "intruders," know that the problem may not be solely a reflection issue but a hallucination.

o o o

Wanders Off

A senior center in Germany had a growing problem: Its residents occasionally would decide they wanted to go "home" or visit relatives and would walk away to look for the nearest bus to take them home.

Solution: Staffers installed a replica of the town's familiar green and yellow bus signs right outside the door, next to a bench. Their long-term memory intact, residents would recognize the distinctive sign and sit down at the "bus stop" to wait. That delayed the wanderers long enough for staffers to find them.

"The bus is delayed," they'd explain. "Would you like to come in for a cup of coffee while you wait?" The residents would come back inside — and promptly forget about their earlier decision to leave.

These phantom bus stops have since popped up in other care homes in the country.

WHY it happens:

At root, people wander because of cognitive changes that cause confusion, disorientation, and other inabilities to recognize what they're doing, where they are, or how to get back.

If your loved one hasn't wandered off yet, prepare yourself as if he will. About 3 out of every 5 people with Alzheimer's wander at some point — that is, they leave home of their own free will but become too confused or lost to make it back home on their own. Usually they're going about normal activities; it's not that they sneak or run away. And if someone disappears once, he's more likely to do so again. Some experts say it can take six to eight episodes before family members recognize a pattern or the danger the behavior poses.

The label "wandering" sounds a lot more pleasant than the experience: Every year older adults with Alzheimer's are found nearly frozen or dehydrated, hit by cars, mugged, or even drowned or otherwise dead after having wandered off. Of those who are not located within 24 hours, half will be seriously or fatally injured, according to the Alzheimer's Association.

Wandering is especially dangerous because people with dementia don't usually think they're lost. So they don't ask for help or directions. They often don't even respond to their own name as searchers call. Some hide instinctively. Others insist, when found, that they're not lost at all — confounding searchers. Police say that 90 percent of wanderers are found within a five-mile radius of where they disappeared.

Someone with dementia may take off due to...

- Habit. Someone used to walking, jogging, or driving may take off as if to do so, only to falter midway — unsure of his location or how to get back. People often leave for "work" at a certain time of day. The sight of a coat on a peg may trigger the habit of putting it on and walking out the door.

- Fear or anxiety. Too much noise (at a party, for example) or a perceived threat may trigger flight.

- A sensation of loss. Someone feeling upset about missing something (literally or figuratively) may wander off to seek it.

- Curiosity. People with Alzheimer's live in the moment. A passing truck, bird, or other distraction can pique interest and the person follows it along. Someone in a new residence may wander off to explore.

TRY this:

To prevent wandering:

- Know the risk factors. People are candidates for wandering and getting lost if they begin to return from normal outings (like walks or drives) later than usual or if they try to "go home" when at home already or to "go to work" when they're retired. Be wary if your loved one seems bored or restless or gets upset in a public space. Not being able to find a public restroom or other common location is another red flag.

If someone with dementia has been late or gone missing at least once:

Consider possible triggers:

- Have there been any big changes in his life? A recent move or a new caregiver, for example, can be stressful. In stressful times, reinforce a comforting routine. Consider making fewer outings.

- Have any medications changed? Agitation could be a side effect; mention the wandering to the prescribing doctor.

- Is there a pattern to the wandering episodes? If it always happens at night, for example, it could indicate fear or loneliness — and he may need extra support after dark. If it's at mealtimes, he may be hungry or thirsty and unable to follow through on these desires. Some people wander at specific times linked to activities from their previous work life or other former routines. Target those times with new, engrossing activities that distract from the impulse to wander.

- Is he busy enough? Ideally, aim for a daily schedule that includes a variety of different activities, outdoor time if he's able, and social time. Having a routine and a full, diverse schedule are two of the best ways to minimize wandering. Being busy by day also makes it more likely he'll sleep through the night.

Create a safe wandering environment, if you can. While this isn't an option for all, if you have a large yard that can be secured, you might be able to set up a place for controlled wandering. Set the yard with winding paths or a labyrinth to pace, for example.

Reduce temptations to wander. Some ideas:

- Keep keys out of sight. Someone who has Alzheimer's

that's severe enough to include wandering shouldn't be driving. But he may still recognize keys left hanging in a familiar place and drive off — even if you don't think he has memories of driving or still knows how.

- Make doors to the outside hard to open. Try plastic grip-style doorknob covers, found in childproofing catalogs or sites. These can be too hard for an older person with dementia to open. Jam sliding doors with a strip of wood in the bottom of the frame.

- Consider changing locks. Any kind of door lock that's different from what your loved one has always used might work because it's hard for someone with cognitive impairment to learn new things. Try a chain lock in a higher-than usual position or a key lock for a door than once had a button lock.

- Disguise dangerous doorways. A gentle alternative to door locks is to lead him away from certain doors with visual cues that convey that the door is something else. Camouflage possibilities include painting the door to match a surrounding wall or hanging a mirror or a poster of scenery (which might be perceived as a window). You can also buy or paint a mural on the door designed to make it look like a bookshelf or pantry shelf. Some families have had success hanging a "Do not enter" or "STOP" sign on an exit door.

- Position a solid black mat in front of doorways. To some people changes in depth perception cause the black square to read like a hole, making them afraid to cross the threshold.

Skip the lectures and logic. Telling your loved one "not to do that again" will be as effective as telling a toddler not to run off — neither has the cognitive capacity to remember the conversation or act on it. Remember that someone who wanders once is likely to wander again. Also:

- Avoid crowds. Crowded situations — shopping malls, big parties, outdoor plazas and events — can produce stress that leads to wandering off not just in that place but even once you're back home. It's also harder for you to keep track of your loved one in a crowd; you can't be distracted for a moment.

- Avoid leaving a wanderer in the car alone. While you're running a quick errand in the bank or drugstore, he's liable to become frightened or worried and slip out of the vehicle.

- Look into alarms that signal movement. You can buy bed pads or chair pads with wireless remote alarms that offer an immediate alert when someone gets up; look for them online. Other devices include floor mats with remote alarms, motion detectors that send alerts directly to a caregiver, and conventional door chimes that sound when a door is opened. Or go low tech: One caregiver hung Christmas bells in such a way that they jingled loudly whenever the door opened.

- Tell immediate neighbors about the Alzheimer's and the person's tendency to wander. Ask them to call you if he uncharacteristically comes over to visit or is seen walking alone.

- Because you can't leave a wanderer home alone safely even for short periods, look into adult day programs or a relief caregiver when you must go out.

- Avoid using restraints. Aside from being inhumane, they've been shown to cause injury. Locking a person with dementia in his room can cause anxiety and aggression that persists for days — and only make him more prone to wander.

- Keep hallways and walking paths inside the living area clear and easy to meander in.

Tip: **"I started to take Dad to the gym with me — he couldn't do that much, but he liked it and the extra activity seemed to wear him out. He slept better and stopped trying to leave the house." — M.C.**

Prepare in advance for not being able to locate a wanderer:

- Enroll in a search program. Sponsored by the Alzheimer's Association, the Medic Alert + Safe Return program is a 24-hour nationwide emergency-response system. You can call an 800-number to activate a search that involves local Alzheimer's Association chapters and local law enforcement. Identification jewelry is provided as part of this service. The Alzheimer's Association also offers programs such as Comfort Zone, which includes the use of GPS technology. Check in with your local police station, as well. Many participate in Project Lifesaver, a program that also uses tracking technology to find lost wanderers. Costs vary by area, and it requires the person to wear a small tracking device.

  Note: You should enroll a family member in a program now, even if there's never been a wandering incident. After *Washington Post* writer Tom Jackman's father went missing, he discovered there was a 10-month wait to get in his local Project Lifesaver. (Jackman's dad, 78, drove from his home in Virginia to Baltimore, until he ran out of gas and was found safe, 20 hours later, without recalling why he'd gone there — a first-time incident.)

- Use identification. Safe return-type programs often provide identification to wear. It's also a good idea to write the name, disease, and your phone number inside the jacket a chronic wanderer wears, as well as on a piece of paper in his wallet.

- Pay attention to the person's wardrobe. It's helpful to searchers if you can identify what your loved one had on. One idea: Pare down a chronic wanderer's wardrobe to multiples that look the same.

- Keep a recent photo handy. Many caregivers avoid

photographing a loved one with Alzheimer's because the disease and age can seem to alter his familiar visage. But an up-to-date portrait will help searchers identify him if he's ever lost.

- Take advantage of GPS technology. Cellphones can be programmed to activate GPS, but many people with Alzheimer's no longer carry phones (or never did), or have outdated models. One option is to wear a phone on a belt or a pair of "smart" shoes containing GPS sensors. (Search online for "Alzheimer's GPS shoe.")

- Consider arranging online bank accounts if you don't have them already. Someone missing can sometimes be traced by credit card spending, but it's most helpful when the accounts are automated.

Tip: **"I got rid of Dad's dark shirts but kept the brightest Aloha-prints he liked, along with his solid orange and yellow polos. That way he was easier to spot when he wandered off." — E.R.**

If someone does go missing...

- Call 911; don't hesitate. Don't wait for the usual "missing for 24 hours" rule of thumb to take effect. Especially in very hot or cold weather, it's best to call for help within 15 minutes. With impaired judgment and memory loss, someone with Alzheimer's who's lost is in harm's way and needs help getting home. In addition to local systems for locating missing older adults with Alzheimer's, the majority of states have Silver Alert systems (public notifications about missing, impaired older adults) that authorities can activate.

- Know where to look. Most who walk (not drive) off are found within a mile of home. In a University of Florida analysis of 675 incidents involving the Alzheimer's Association Safe Return program, one fourth of wanderers turned up in a residential yard. About one fifth were found standing in streets. Others turned up at senior centers, restaurants, shopping centers, and other businesses.

Other studies have shown that wanderers often are found in ditches and creeks and behind bushes and briars, usually not far from a road. Two-thirds cross a road at some point.

To help you cope:

- Try not to take wandering as a criticism of your care. Wandering is rarely an attempt to "escape" a disliked situation; that would involve more premeditation and planning than most people with Alzheimer's are capable of. The relatives of good, loving, and attentive caregivers still wander.

o o o

SEXUALITY-RELATED PROBLEMS

Makes Inappropriate Advances

"Shari, baby! Where've you been? Your knockers are calling me!" the man said, wiggling his fingers as he reached toward his attractive visitor's breasts.

"Dad! I'm not Sharon, um, Mom. I'm Sue, your daughter," she replied, jumping back.

Her father looked confused for a second. "Well then how about a kiss?"

Sue approached her father for a hug, quickly turning her cheek in case he gave her the wrong kind of kiss.

WHY it happens:

Many people with dementia still have sexual urges — and want to act on them. But with poor impulse control and self-censorship, and lacking the ability to read a social situation as they once did, these feelings can lead someone to behave in ways considered socially wrong.

Advances can range from suggestive comments to propositioning, and from flirtatious touches to groping. Anyone can be a target for the advances: a caregiver, a daughter, an old friend, a virtual stranger. The advances seldom reveal some long-simmering desire now being acted on (as caregivers often believe). Your husband with Alzheimer's making a pass at your old friend of 30 years isn't proof of his secret crush or a past affair, for example, and shouldn't be taken that way. The target is usually someone who's handy out of sheer proximity.

Sometimes a parent mistakes an adult child for his or her spouse, leading to awkward moments. The person with dementia isn't thinking incest, of course; he really believes the adult child is someone else. Bathing is a common trigger. Sexual inappropriateness can also be a bid for attention.

Disinhibition (lack of self control) about sex is thought to affect up to one in four people with dementia. Men and women are about equally affected, according to a 2005 article in the British journal, *Advances in Psychiatric Treatment*, although sexual complaints about men are more common. For unknown reasons (possibly better reporting but also the sheer number of people living together), it's more often seen in nursing homes. This behavior can increase as the disease progresses before finally subsiding in late-stage Alzheimer's.

Things that can contribute include a lack of a regular partner (such as in a widower who develops dementia), boredom, or misinterpreting cues seen on TV or overheard. People who struggled to contain hypersexual behavior when they were healthy often behave inappropriately now. Delirium, a behavior syndrome caused by a physical stress such as an infection or pain, can also cause sexually inappropriate behavior.

TRY this:

- If the behavior is sudden and new, consider a medical evaluation to rule out delirium or related causes. .

- If the behavior is ongoing, see if you can identify and remove a trigger for the behavior. Is it always directed to a particular person? (If it's an aide, for example, you might need to make a staff change.) Does it happen on days the routine is disrupted? When the person drinks? During help with personal care?

- Make sure he isn't drinking too much. Alcohol can add to disinhibition in someone with dementia just as in someone with a healthy brain.

- Try not to shame the person or make him feel embarrassed. Act as neutrally as you can muster.

- Restate your relationship: "Hi, Dad, it's your #1 daughter and fan, Sue!" "Look: Mrs. Smith, the hairdresser, has come to trim your hair."

- Gently but firmly set a boundary. "That's not how we say hello." "Please don't talk that way, okay?"

Tip: " **My sister-in-law used humor with my dad (her father-in-law): 'You old devil! You know I'm a married woman, so please stop, or Jack might beat you up! '"** — K. S.

- Respond quickly with distraction to get his mind off sexual activity. Find a fresh activity or move to a different room. Offering a snack can satisfy a different kind of physical craving.

- Avoid friendly flirtatiousness or sexual-type teasing, which might be misinterpreted. At the same time, some people will act less sexually if they have increased platonic physical affection — hand holding, hugs, even walking arm in arm or dancing together. You have to see what works in your specific case.

- If helping with bathing is a trigger, have someone of the same sex handle this task.

- Strange but true creative solutions: A 68-year-old man with dementia in one facility turned his advances to a three-foot-tall Pink Panther doll and stopped trying to molest staff, according to a report in the *American Journal of Geriatric Psychiatry*. The soft proportions of a body pillow might also comfort someone long accustomed to having a bed partner.

- If the problem is severe, mention it to a doctor. Other strategies should always be tried first because there's not good research on using medications to treat the problem, and drugs can have unwanted side effects. Meds that can be used to treat sexual disinhibition include antiandrogens (hormone treatment that impairs sexual functioning), mood stabilizers, antidepressants, and antipsychotics (a last-resort drug for people with dementia because they can cause other problems).

To help you cope:

- Know that for an adult child, this can be one of the more distressing problems to deal with — especially when you're the target of the unwanted advances. The mix of shock, distaste, guilt, and confusion you may feel is absolutely normal. It's the ultimate muddling of your social roles.

- Some caregivers find talking to a counselor or therapist helpful — not because they've done anything amiss, but to gain perspective and coping advice.

- Remind friends and visitors who are targeted that the disease is causing this behavior. Some caregivers report losing "shocked" friends over this, but more typical is for people to be deeply empathetic. If a friend grows reluctant to visit in person, try to schedule visits when your loved one is asleep or when there's back-up help, as it's also important for you to have time with friends.

o o o

Makes Unwanted Advances to Spouse

Cora has begun to dread evening — and bedtime. She and Stanislaus, her husband of 57 years, have a good marriage and she still loves him. But his sex drive is still strong, and increasingly, this troubles her.

"In the first few years after he was diagnosed, when we were intimate was like being with the old Stan; he seemed fine," she says. "But as he's become more child-like and needs more help from me, I just don't like thinking of him that way [sexually] any more. It makes me uncomfortable."

WHY it happens:

We're sexual beings. The instinct and habit that make up our sexuality are deeply rooted. People with early stage dementia continue to become aroused and have desire. Many couples find intimate time to be a source of mutual comfort and reassurance at a turbulent time. Your loved one may even seem more like his or her "old self" during sex.

For many couples, though, the desire to have sex dissipates early in the disease process, especially on the side of the caregiving spouse, and these feelings of disconnection grow as the disease progresses. The partner's increasing dependency changes the way they view their intimate relationship and makes desire wane. Stress and exhaustion take a toll, too. Some mates say they feel like they're "giving" something to a confused partner who expresses desire, even though they themselves are no longer sexually attracted. More commonly, caregiving mates grow turned off by cognitive changes and wrestle with guilt or sexual frustration. Still other caregiving spouses believe sex under later-stage circumstances is unethical because their loved one is incapable of fully understanding what he's doing. (Indeed, some people with dementia become frightened or upset by advances made toward them.)

Should you? Shouldn't you? What's right? "There are a lot more questions than answers," says geriatric psychiatrist Ken Robbins. The "right" answer to what one's sex life looks like after a dementia diagnosis is completely personal.

TRY this:

In general:

- Ask yourself what your partner would think if your positions were reversed. Do you still feel sex is a marital "duty" if you aren't interested and your partner is impaired? What does your conscience tell you? It's an entirely individual call, but those kinds of questions can be a useful tool to think things through.

- Consider talking to a therapist if you're conflicted, distressed, or sad. A neutral third party can help you sort out your feelings.

In the moment:

- If you're not comfortable having sex, make up a white lie. Caregiver advocate Carol D. O'Dell, author of *Mothering Mother*, recommends telling a fib about why you can't right now. Your partner may quickly forget when the urge passes.

- Substitute other nonsexual forms of giving physical affection, such as a shoulder rub or holding hands. It may be enough to satisfy the person's need for touch and reassurance.

- Use distraction. Change activities to something absorbing (a car ride, playing with a pet). Or offer a favorite snack: "Let's have a cookie first."

To help you cope:

- Even when a sexual relationship falters, couples can still feel intimacy. Talking, touching, hand-holding, spending time together, and just knowing that you're there seeing your partner through his or her chronic illness can reinforce close feelings.

- Consider separate sleeping arrangements. You don't have to make a big deal about it, but let it evolve. One caregiving spouse stayed up later each night and would go to another room to sleep; her husband, a sound sleeper, didn't notice, and she'd awaken first.

What About Sex Outside Your Marriage?

Support groups and others report rising numbers of Alzheimer's caregivers contemplating sexual relationships outside of marriage. Given that Alzheimer's can be a long disease, and many partners are still in their prime sexual years themselves, especially in the rising numbers of early-onset cases, the math can be daunting. Obviously this is a controversial decision, with many considerations. Some believe the vow of "til death do us part" means that the well partner should hang tough for the duration, period. Others believe that marriage vows are made between two parties of sound mind, but that pledges should be allowed to change when one of those minds becomes unsound.

This is one dilemma, caregivers consistently say, where those who haven't experienced Alzheimer's firsthand might hold their tongues before weighing in with an opinion. Companionship changes. Sharing changes. A relationship rocked by Alzheimer's is no longer equal or reciprocal. The loss of the sexual dimension of a long, happy partnership can layer more stress and sadness on the healthy spouse who's already grappling with so many losses. These are incalculably tough things to come to terms with. (And if the partnership wasn't happy, that adds another troubling factor in the mix.)

As Richard Anderson, past-president of the Well Spouse Association puts it, "the emotional well being of both partners is paramount."

Ultimately it's a decision only you and your conscience can make.

What helps:

- Talk to a trusted therapist or clergyperson. (Know that clergy have come down on both sides of this ethical dilemma.) Beware of input from friends, who may have trouble separating their own personal agendas from your dilemma or may not be able to fully relate.

- Realize that adult children often take issue with such a relationship. They may be grappling with denial about the Alzheimer's or not want to think too closely about their parents' intimate relationship. They may have some unrelated, unresolved issue with a parent that colors their view. In the end, though, your sex life isn't their business now any more than it ever was.

o o o

Masturbates Publicly

Mary Jo began to avoid bringing her kids to visit Grandpa Joe. One day, she left them all watching cartoons together in the family room while she made sandwiches in the kitchen with her mom. When she poked her head in the room to call them all to lunch, she saw "Grandpa Joe" sitting in his recliner with his hands in his pants.

"The kids didn't notice, but I was mortified," she says. "I don't know what set him off — something in the cartoon, or what. Maybe he does that all the time, but I was too embarrassed to even ask my mom about it."

WHY it happens:

As with making inappropriate advances, this kind of sexual behavior happens because people with dementia lose the ability to judge what's socially acceptable. They may act on impulse more and lack self-control (disinhibition).

Sometimes people with dementia who masturbate actually have to use the toilet. They may fumble with their clothes for that reason and then forget the need to urinate and fondle themselves instead.

Examples of related behaviors: undressing in public, purposely exposing one's self, and using pornography (magazines, videos) when others are present.

TRY this:

- If the behavior is recent and new, have him evaluated for delirium, urinary tract infection, prostate trouble, or another treatable physical cause.

- See if you can identify a trigger — a person, situation, or time of day — that seems to set off the behavior.

- Keep calm to avoid shaming, which can cause other problems.

- Escort him to a private place. If it's his bedroom or bathroom, say, "You can only do that in here."

- Distract with an offer of a snack or something else to do.

- Provide hands-on activities at times when the masturbation typically occurs; working with the hands can be an effective distraction and deterrent.

- Look into clothing that's more difficult to remove, such as dressing a man in overalls without a front fly.

- If the problem is severe, mention it to a doctor. Other strategies should always be tried first because there's not good research on using medications to treat the problem, and drugs can have unwanted side effects. Meds that may be used to treat sexual disinhibition include antiandrogens (hormone treatment that impairs sexual functioning), mood stabilizers, antidepressants, and antipsychotics (a last-resort drug for people with dementia because they can cause other problems).

o o o

COMMUNICATION PROBLEMS

Can't Find the Right Words

Zelda stood in front of her daughter with her hands on her hips. "Where's my — my — my — my read."

"Read?" her daughter, Zoe, asked, blankly.

"Box! Read box. You know, my read box! I just had it."

"Breadbox?"

Zelda shook her head. "Of course not, silly! You know what I mean!"

"Mom, I don't. Read box? You mean like a Kindle? You don't have one, Mom. Do you want an e-reader?"

Zelda finally spotted her paperback book on the kitchen table. "Oh, here it is."

WHY it happens:

Trouble finding the right word is a common early sign of Alzheimer's, since both memory and parts of the brain used for speech and language are affected. This is also called *aphasia* or *primary progressive aphasia* (PPA). PPA is considered a symptom of dementia often seen with Alzheimer's. (Not everyone with Alzheimer's has it.)

PPA gets progressively worse, although the rate of decline is different for each person. It affects not only word choice but also the ability to speak clearly, understand others, read, and write. Some people have trouble in one of these areas but not others. At first, for example, your loved one may have trouble finding words but reasoning and visual perception involved with reading and writing are still intact. Spelling and math problems (such as writing numerals or adding them) are related effects.

Aphasia is also common with stroke victims; those who also have vascular dementia (caused by small strokes or blood vessel disease) may show this symptom.

What you might hear:

- Hesitancy and long pauses in the middle of a sentence as the person searches for the word

- A generic term substituted for any word, such as *thingamabob, stuff, thingy, that-there* (*white stuff* for salt, *black stuff* for pepper)

- Substitution of a word or phrase that's somehow related (so *read box* for book, *writing stick* for pencil, *mouth cleaner* for toothbrush)

- Substitution of a similar-sounding word or made-up word (*kappy* for kitty, *launch* for lunch, *sweer* for shower)

- Getting stuck on a word and repeating it over and over

- Stringing together lots of nonsense words or gibberish

- Words whispered or spoken so softly that you can barely hear them, much less make them out

- You might also notice that someone who has trouble speaking may still be able to understand what's said to her.

TRY this:

- Don't get caught up in trying to "teach" her the correct word or make a big deal about the mistake. Sometimes the goofs are pretty funny, but laugh only if self-deprecating humor or lightness is part of your loved one's personality. Otherwise you'll risk embarrassing her.

- Early on, give her some space to come up with the right word. If you rush in to supply it, she may feel edgy. If she's really foundering, wait a few seconds, then go ahead and supply what you think she means. "Oh, your book? It's on your chair."

- Make it your problem. Social worker and Alzheimer's expert Joyce Simard often blames herself when asking someone to repeat. "I'm sorry, my hearing isn't so good. What did you say?"

- Pay attention to gesturing and body language, as well as the context of the rest of the sentence, to discern meaning.

Tip: **"Mom took to carrying around a notebook in which she'd write down questions or comments for us. She had a lot of trouble talking, but early on, she could still write, and it eased her frustration." —J.R.**

- Speak slowly, and focus on getting just one idea across at a time. ("Let's eat lunch," not "After lunch we'll go to the store for your art supplies.")

- Try exposing the person to arts such as music or painting. Some research shows that those whose language capacity shrinks often enjoy creative outlets they never had (or even showed an interest in) before, as a means of self-expression.

- Consider visiting a speech pathologist or occupational therapist who has experience working with dementia patients. Especially early in the disease, or if the person has also had a stroke, they can often help find new ways to communicate.

- Create "I have aphasia cards" to discreetly hand out in public. The National Stroke Association recommends carrying cards that say something like, "My mother has aphasia, which means she can't speak well or understand speech well. Please speak clearly and slowly. Thanks for your patience."

To help you cope:

- Your patience may be sorely tested because these speech changes can be maddening, confusing, and even scary. But getting upset will only make your loved one upset.

Realize that this is a very frustrating and frightening development for your loved one, too. Reach out with added hugs, physical contact, and supportiveness to help her feel more loved and connected despite the wedge of a language barrier.

o o o

Uses Nonsense Words, Gibberish

"Hey diddlie diddle, do do do do," Lucille croons to herself as she rocks in her usual armchair. "Do do majig."

"How are you today, Mama?" asks her husband, Bill. They've been married for 63 years.

"Diddlie diddle. I want my majiggy jig," Lucille responds.

Bill has no idea what she's saying. "Yes, love, I'm going to make our lunch right now with your favorite brownies for dessert," he says. He kisses the top of her head as he passes by.

WHY it happens:

Language that doesn't make sense is an extreme kind of aphasia — or loss of language — caused by dementia. This particular loss tends to show up in moderate or late dementia. She's lost the ability to find the right words and express them.

Speech may be a mix of nonsense words and a few that make sense, garbled-sounding real speech, or purely nonsensical.

This speech pattern can also become an almost involuntary self-soothing habit. She calms herself down through this kind of talk. Some people only use nonsense speech when tired and trying to sleep.

TRY this:

- Avoid urging someone with this problem to try to be clearer. She literally can't try any harder.

- Read body language to see if it can help you figure out a meaning.

- See if you can connect a mood to the speech, either through the tone used or the circumstances. Someone who can't find something or doesn't want to go somewhere might mutter angrily, for example.

- Show added love and reassurance if the gibberish seems to increase when your loved one is upset, lonely, or bored.

To help you cope:

- Listening to gibberish can get a bit stressful and make a loved one seem remote from you. But don't worry too much about exactly interpreting what she's trying to say. Stick to a routine and try to anticipate needs (time to be hungry for lunch?).

o o o

Asks, "What Should I Be Doing?"

An aide wheels my mother-in-law into the sunny dining room where she lives with her husband and my sister-in-law and her family. It's a holiday, and everyone's just sitting around, relaxed.

"How are you today?" someone asks.

"I'm fine," she assures. "What should I be doing?"

"You don't need to do anything, Mom," her daughter tells her. "Paula and Jim are here visiting, and we're going to have lunch soon."

"Oh, okay." Then, a few minutes later she asks her husband: "What should I be doing? Is there something I should be doing?" — P.S.S.

WHY it happens:

Humans have an inborn need to be busy, to contribute. This feeling is especially strong among those who have been active all their lives, working and/or looking after others. At the same time, loving, well-meaning family caregivers tend to want to make life easy for the person with Alzheimer's. We do as much as we can for them. Sometimes, that's too much.

Without a task or responsibility to manage, a child to raise, a job to tend, your loved one may have little or nothing to do. Yet she still feels a lingering sensation that she *should* be doing something. (Feelings tend to live longer and stronger than memories.) It's like that haunting feeling you get when you walk into a room intending to do something, but once you're there, you can't put your finger on what it was.

Confusion, boredom, and anxiety can bring these feelings to the fore. When she's frail and unable to do much, the problem is intensified.

TRY this:

- Look for ways to involve the person in meaningful activities. Even the smallest acts, or things you'll wind up having to re-do later, can fill the bill. The definition of "meaningful" will change over time as mental and physical abilities change. It doesn't have to be much to provide the satisfying feelings of contributing.

- Consider making one or two special tasks her designated chore. You'll want to match the task to her ability, but taking ownership of something can underscore a sense of purpose. Maybe your mom always sets the table or folds the laundry. Maybe your dad brings in the mail (if wandering isn't a potential issue).

- Remind yourself to ask for her help. We all love to be sought after and included. Ask her help when tying a ribbon on a package or stirring a soup. Or simply solicit her opinion on whether the soup needs salt or which color of ribbon looks best on the gift you're wrapping.

- Focus on what she can do now, not what she once did. Say your mom can no longer bake her special oatmeal cookies. But perhaps she can "coach" you in the steps (even though she may not remember them and you'll be the one guiding her along). Or you can give her slice-and-bake dough to form on cookie sheets, a familiar act.

- Don't worry about programming every minute of the day, but do try to weave some interesting activities into your daily routine. This stamps out boredom and brings purpose to the day.

o o o

Curses (But Didn't Used to) or Says Other Mean, Hurtful, or Inappropriate Things

"You cheap SOB!" Elizabeth raged at Frank, her husband of 49 years. "Why don't you buy me some new clothes, you f——ing bastard!" For most of her life, the elegant and well-bred Elizabeth was soft-spoken and unfailingly polite. Frank always admired how she knew just the right thing to say in any circumstance.

"The first time she cursed, she said "dammit" under her breath when she was having trouble getting out of the car," Frank says. "That alone was kind of shocking. But I figured it was because she was upset by her Alzheimer's diagnosis." Then she began hurling swear words behind his back, often when she didn't want to do something he asked her to do — take a bath, eat dinner, go to bed. As the years went on the sailor-talk became louder — and more frequent. Mostly, these outbursts have been targeted at poor Frank.

"She has all the clothes she could want, I'm gentle, I don't deny her anything," he says with sadness. "She makes up a lot of indignities and hurls the most horrible words at me — words I never knew she'd even heard!"

WHY it happens:

Swearing is rarely intentional in someone who has dementia, especially when it's a new behavior for the person. It's surprisingly common, though, for mild-mannered people to begin using salty phrases they never before uttered.

A healthy person might *think* something crude when angry but not voice it. We're taught not to do so as children, and these messages are reinforced by the norms of polite society. As adults, we then automatically self-censor things we know not to be appropriate. In dementia, however, there's damage to the part of the brain's processing centers involved in self-control. The person becomes less able to regulate certain behaviors, including language.

Swearing is often triggered by anger, frustration, or fear.

Interestingly, there's research to show that even in healthy people, occasional cursing is a way to cut the sensation of pain.

The loss of self-control in dementia (called disinhibition) can also cause someone to use uncharacteristically crude words, belch or pass gas loudly, holler nonsense, wail, make random animal sounds, or say rude comments. (One caregiver reports his wife would make a low "moo" sound whenever she saw an obese person in public.)

TRY this:

- At first, try drawing a line: "Please don't talk to me like that, Jane." "That's not a very nice word." Then distract to another activity or conversation. But if the chiding doesn't work and the cursing continues, simply ignore it.

- Avoid dramatic shushing or shaming. Try not to act shocked or startled. It can make someone with dementia feel bad or even fuel more of the behavior, without solving the problem. Better: React with calm indifference.

- Look for an underlying trigger: Is she feeling stressed? Bored? Upset about something? Is it too noisy, for example, or are children speaking faster than the person with dementia can understand? Addressing the cause of the emotion can often end a bout of potty mouth.

- One way to find a trigger is to look for patterns. Does the meanness tend to come out at certain times, such as during bathing? Maybe there's something about the experience that is upsetting, like your loved one is getting chilled without your realizing it. Bob DeMarco, the founder of Alzheimer's Reading Room, noticed his mother would hurl hurtful language his way whenever he'd been talking on the phone. He eventually figured out that she believed he was talking to someone about putting her in a "home," one of her fears. Long detailed explanations that this wasn't true were of no use. What worked: Being extra loving and reassuring with hugs and words after he hung up, then distracting with a pleasant activity.

- In public, you can apologetically and discreetly explain that the cursing is an unfortunate behavior caused by her dementia. Some families have business cards made to (again, discreetly) hand to wait staff, store clerks, or others in public settings: "Please excuse my [wife/mother]; she has dementia, which causes her to act in unpredictable ways."

- If children overhear, explain to them that, "Grandma has a sickness in her brain that makes her talk funny and say bad words. She never used them before she got sick, and you shouldn't either."

- Mention a tough case to the doctor. Certain medications or drug interactions can increase disinhibition in some people.

To help you cope:

- Let yourself grieve. This behavior can be distressing to witness and endure.

- Don't make the common mistake of assuming the epithets are the affected person's "real personality" or "true feelings about you" coming out. Even if the swearing is directed at you personally, it's usually a response to how she's feeling in the moment about something going on.

- Know that using vulgar language can be one of those intractable behaviors where the best you can do is to "grin and bear it." Some caregivers use humor to cut the discomfort: "Oh Bess, you sound like someone in an R-rated movie!"

o o o

Says, "I Want to Go Home"

As my grandmother's Alzheimer's progressed, she'd sit in a quiet stupor for most of our visits to the nursing home. She'd moved there two years earlier, after breaking a hip at age 97. At some point, some days, she'd suddenly perk up: "Are we going home? Where's my purse? Have we paid yet?"

She seemed to think we were in a restaurant. And we'd all freeze, unsure what to say. "Gram, this isn't Red Lobster," would only confuse her. So did explaining that this was her home. (I tried that once and she said, "Like hell.") Usually she'd just get adamant: "Bring me my purse; I'm ready to go home now." — P.S.S.

Why it happens

In the language of Alzheimer's, "going home" usually expresses a desire for security. Home is a warm, fuzzy, happy concept for most of us, a place of refuge and nurturing. Think of the expressions, "home is where the heart is," "hearth and home," "home sweet home." Also, memories held the longest are those of earlier life; these are often happy memories of growing up or of a beloved community.

The person with dementia may be feeling some kind of discomfort, and longing for the security that "home" represents. Maybe she's confused because she doesn't recognize where she is (whether it's her own longtime residence, a new care community, or a temporary stay at a hospital). She may be anxious about something (a visit she senses is coming to an end, an upcoming shower or bed bath). Some people also talk about going home when they're tired.

TRY this:

- Skip trying to orient the person by saying, "But you are home!" or "This is your home now." The intellectual capacity to reason is gone. Trying to re-orient will likely lead to more confusion or argument.

- Hear *home* as a feeling your loved one needs you to

understand. Too often someone with dementia is told "you *are* home," but the underlying emotional need goes unaddressed. So the person grows more distressed.

- Instead, try hearing "I want to go home" as "I'm uneasy" or "I'm scared." Try meeting the emotional need — fear, uncertainty — with an upbeat little fib that meets the person where she is, while reassuring: "The weather's too cold now, maybe later." "Why don't we listen to some music first?" Some people with dementia believes they're at a hotel, restaurant, cruise ship, or other trip-related setting, and caregivers go along with this idea: "We'll go back home soon, maybe tomorrow." "A fib-let is better than a tablet," says caregiver advocate and former spousal caregiver Joanne Koenig Coste, author of *Learning to Speak Alzheimer's.*

- Offer reassurance in the form of a hug. Body language is often effective where words and logic won't work. Your loved one wants to feel secure.

- Use verbal reinforcement. At random times, say things like, "I feel so safe and happy living in this nice house." (Avoid saying it in direct argument to, "I want to go home," though.)

- Pay attention to care circumstances that might be triggering the discomfort. Does the person talk about going home at certain times, such as before bedtime? Is there something distressing about her routine at this time (for example, does she dislike showering or have a new care aide who makes her uncomfortable)? This expression isn't necessarily a condemnation of a living situation, but it's worth double-checking for possible problems. Many can be easily fixed and improve your loved one's quality of life.

- Don't bend over backward making a "Trip to Bountiful" reunion visit to a home place. Remember, someone with dementia rarely means *home* literally. She may be thinking of a place she lived in a long time ago, such as her birthplace or the house where she raised her family. Or all the happy places she's lived may be co-mingling in her mind to represent a vague, satisfying feeling, not an actual place. While such a trip can be fun (if she's physically capable), you have to brace for the possibility that even a visit to an intact old home won't satisfy the longing that's been expressed. If the place is gone or altered, even if your loved one can remember it, she may be even more confused.

- If she is insistent about getting in the car or "going now," try this. Go for a drive (such as around the block or out for ice cream). Pull back up to her current residence and cheerfully announce, "We're home!"

- Use *home* as a springboard for distracting conversation. "You really miss home. Tell me about it." Ask about favorite activities or places "back home" or what she'll do first when she "gets home."

- Go *home* with photos. Look at old pictures from the stage of life about which the person seems to have happy memories. Don't do it intending to orient: "See, this is your home! The old one was burned down, remember?" Instead, do it as a way to placate: "We can't go home yet, but look at these pictures I found. Let's look at them and plan our trip."

To help you cope....

- Separate your emotions from what's being said. Hearing, "I want to go home," can provoke many feelings: worry that a loved one is unhappy in a given setting; guilt at having made an out-of-home placement; disappointment or anger that she sounds unsatisfied by all the sacrifices you're making on her behalf. Those who have taken in an adult parent may fear that it means they haven't done enough to make the parent feel at home. Keep in mind that by mid-stage Alzheimer's, when this expression is most used, someone with dementia isn't likely to be saying such things as jibes to manipulate you. Try not to take it personally.

o o o

PERSONAL CARE PROBLEMS

Dislikes Bathing or Won't Bathe

"I'm not dirty! I'm not dirty!" Hal insists whenever his wife, Evelyn, asks if he wants to get in the shower first. She tries to ignore the fact that her once-fastidious husband hasn't bathed or showered in days. She playfully wipes any bits of food from his face after meals, and she makes sure his hair is cut regularly so it doesn't get oily and matted. But after a week or two, she can't ignore the body odor any more.

Sometimes, Hal surprises her by hopping under the running water when she asks. Other times, half the day goes by trying to cajole him into cleaning up.

WHY it happens:

Because bathing is a deeply held habit, someone with Alzheimer's at first remembers to do it. But gradually the sequence of steps may become too difficult to manage. Avoiding it altogether may become easier.

Often other factors contribute to a refusal to bathe:

- Discomfort. Maybe the water is too cold or too hot. Maybe the air temperature varies too much. It's also stressful to stay balanced while trying to not slip.

- Water! It's common for people with dementia to dislike the feeling of water over the face and head.

- Pain. A frail person might find the whole business physically overwhelming.

- Modesty. Being helped by someone of the opposite gender — even a spouse — can make a bather feel self conscious, shy, or deeply embarrassed.

- Dignity. Bathing is personal. Having to be helped represents neediness and makes people feel juvenile or even disrespected, especially when help is provided in a brusque or insensitive way, or invades personal space in

194

an abrupt way.

- Defensiveness. The more you nag, the more a reluctant bather may dig in. It's easier to do nothing.

- Fear. Fear of falling is common. One bad experience — a slip, a rough helper, being chilled — can also be a turn-off because he's wary of repeating the experience. The incident itself may be forgotten, but the sound of water running or the sight of the tub remains vaguely agitating.

TRY this:

To encourage bathing:

- Start by reinforcing a routine. Bathing should happen at the same time every day — ideally, not when it's most convenient for you or a helper but when and how he always did it. (First thing in the morning? After a walk? Before bed. Shower or bath? Soap or bath gel?)

- Avoid asking how long it's been since the last shower or talking about how much it's needed. Just start preparations.

- Get as many things ready in advance as possible. Heat up the room to a comfortable temperature. Have toiletries and towels ready. If you have to leave your loved one alone to retrieve something, he may give up and leave.

- Try leading the person to a prepared bath — as if you were walking somewhere else — without talking about it. The idea isn't to surprise but to minimize hesitation. Then mention the benefits: "You always like that clean, calm feeling after your bath. See if the water temperature feels good to you."

- Try spilling a little juice or sauce on a reluctant bather. "Oh, look what I did! Let me help you out of that...well, since you're changing, how about a quick bath, so you won't have to bother later."

Tip: "I would tell Mom, 'Remember that smell Dad got

when he'd get dirty? I think you're starting to have some of that and I know you wouldn't want that. It's hard to smell on your own self, I know. Maybe today would be a nice day for a bath.'" — A.K.

- Go bit-by-bit. Say, "How about we just get your feet wet?" Stress how relaxing it feels. Once the shoes and socks are off and the feet washed, try hands next. Then say you'd like to wash the arms, then the back. Cover what you've just cleaned with a dryer-warmed towel. Starting with one body part at a time can often coax someone through a complete sponge bath.

- Give the person being bathed a washcloth to hold, even if he isn't capable any more of doing the work. That keeps the hands busy and feels "right." Encourage someone who's able to clean to do as much as possible — don't do it all for him.

To increase comfort:

- Help the person associate bathing with positive feelings by making it as pleasant an experience as possible. With time and patience, this approach can also turnaround someone who's skittish because of a previous bad experience.

- Employ distractions. Set up a music player and play soft big band music or jazz. A sports fan might like to listen to a game on the radio. Consider a lava lamp, a portable TV, or fish bowl to look at if there's room and it's safe.

- Try warming towels and robe in the dryer for 10 minutes during a bath, before they're needed. They'll retain warmth and feel cozy.

- Install a bath bench (available at medical supply stores or some drugstores). Being seated can raise a sense of security in the shower or make sponge baths easier in the tub. Secure grab bars are also worth the small investment.

- Use a hand-held shower nozzle. It's easier to control the flow of water, and you can keep it away from the face and hair.

- For someone struggling with modesty, use small towels to cover genitals and breasts and wash underneath them.

- Avoid using bath oils, which can make skin slippery and hard to hold.

- Keep up a patter of conversation — talk about a TV show plot or news about relatives — anything that distracts from the personal nature of what you're doing.

- Cover the mirror. Around moderate-stage dementia, a reflection or movement noticed within it can be perceived as a stranger "watching." This can raise inhibition.

- Options for washing hair: Some bathers find a scalp massage during shampooing a delight, especially if you take care to keep water out of the face with a hand-nozzle and a washcloth to cover the eyes. Others enjoy dry shampoo products. You can also wash hair using a washcloth: Dab on a small amount of shampoo and rinse out with a clean wet cloth. Another option: Leave hair washing to be part of a weekly salon or barbershop appointment instead of doing it at home.

- Find the right pace. If you go too slow, he may get chilled. Go too fast, and he'll feel rushed and irritated.

To help you cope....

- Reconsider frequency. A daily bath probably isn't necessary if the habit has been lost. Try a daily "top and tail" (face and genitals) and a weekly bath.

- If he's just too resistant or if you're having any kind of physical trouble (such as a bad back or trying to help someone bigger than you), try hiring a home aide of the same gender as your loved one to come just once a week, or several times a week, for bathing. If professional help isn't in the cards, maybe there's a family member better suited to the task who can take it on — a son to help a father, for example.

o o o

Dressing: Chooses Inappropriate Clothes

As her dementia progressed, my mother-in-law's favorite outfit seemed to be a navy tracksuit made of heavy fleece. It was a little different from the smart sweaters, trousers, and coordinating jewelry she'd always worn. But I could see the appeal: It was easy to put on and off, and comfortable.

One hot summer day, arriving for a visit, we were knocked over by a wave of heat when opening the garage door. The air-conditioning in her house was broken. It was 95 degrees. But Louie was wearing her usual fleece tracksuit. It had become her go-to uniform — winter or summer, air conditioning or no air conditioning. — P.S.S.

WHY it happens:

Loss of judgment and decision-making ability leave someone unable to weigh factors like weather, season, and occasion, and make sensible choices. It's complicated for any of us to figure out the appropriate thing to wear each day. For someone with dementia, this can lead to lots of mix-ups, like light jackets in blizzards, sequins at the local diner, or sporting gear at church.

Clothing involves many parts to coordinate and assemble, adding to the challenge. Many people get overwhelmed by the options.

TRY this:

- Simplify the choices. Pare down the closet and drawers, so they contain a limited number of appropriate options.

- Change out closets with the seasons. Make sure the only choices that are accessible suit the season. Store bulky sweaters in boxes in another room during the summer, for example. Get rid of bathing suits, evening wear, and business suits that are never worn.

- Lay out the next day's outfits. Layer them in the order they're to be put on — so underclothes are on top, above shirts and pants.

- Make sure all the clothes are easy-on, easy-off. Most

people find success with elastic waistbands, popover ponchos, loose sweaters, cardigans with zippers, tube socks without heels, and Velcro-strap shoes.

o o o

Dressing: Wears the Same Clothes Over and Over

My father had always been a careful dresser. After he retired from his life of white shirts and ties, he wore a full rainbow of golf shirts and owned more cardigans than Mister Rogers. But if you'd met him late in his dementia, you'd invariably see him in a stained plaid shirt and baggy, wrinkled gray trousers — day after day after day.

"The worst part was trying to wash them," recalls my sister-in-law. "He wouldn't put them in the hamper. He hung them up and put them on again in the morning before I could sneak in and get them away." — P.S.S.

Why it happens

Impaired short-term memory causes someone with dementia to forget the clothes are dirty as soon as they undress. Impaired judgment means that the usual clues (stained, wrinkled, smelly) don't add up to the usual response (put them in the hamper to be washed).

Donning the same handy clothes the next day can be easier than having to choose among many clothes in drawers or the closet. Making choices can be cognitively overwhelming. Familiarity, in contrast, is comforting.

TRY this:

- Steer clear of logic, such as pointing out, "Honestly, Dad! You wore the same outfit yesterday!" Not only is it hard for someone with dementia to follow logic but you risk putting him on the defensive and setting up a no-win argument.

- When he's sound asleep, go in his room to remove the dirty clothes. Lay out something similar in the same spot. As long as replacement clothes are handy in the morning, he's apt to forget about the dirty favorite. If he should notice, make a big fuss over a white lie: "Oh Dad! I'm so sorry! I spilled juice on your favorite shirt

201

yesterday and nearly ruined it! I've sent it to the cleaners, but meanwhile I found this one. Oh, I hope you can forgive me!"

- If the person prefers having the old clothes hung back up at day's end, help him do so. Keep the dirty clothes to one side of the closet, so you know which they are and can wash them later. Put clean clothes in a more prominent place.

- Pare down the closet, so there are far fewer options (just a few shirts, for example), which can make choosing clean clothes easier. Bonus: If you make sure everything matches, there will be no more clashing outfits. Choose solids in a favorite color over patterns, which can be distracting and irritating to someone with dementia.

- Buy identical multiple versions of favorites, so one set can be washed while the other is worn. Bonus: Only one type of sock, for example, means no more mismatches.

- If your loved one sleeps in the same clothes, your only chance may be to take them away for washing when he bathes. Bring clean clothes into the bathroom to put on afterward. You may have to settle for a change of clothes only every few days if he won't bathe daily.

To help you cope:

- Make sure the real problem is dirt and odor, not your own irritation by the repetition of the outfit. A few generations ago, nobody changed clothes every day.

o o o

Dental-Care Trouble

One day Vicki was startled to see her husband, Charles, brushing his teeth — with the wrong end of the toothbrush. "What are you doing?" she asked.

"What does it look like?!"

"You're holding the brush upside down!" she told him.

Charles stared at the brush for a second. "I knew that!" he said, putting it down quickly. After that incident, Vicki began to notice that the toothbrush went unused for days.

WHY it happens:

Oral-care problems are common in people with dementia. This is such a central part of private self care that caregivers sometimes forget about it. We just expect that it's being taken care of, until bad breath, tooth pain, or other problems crop up.

Some people simply forget to brush (or take care of dentures). Others begin having trouble with the steps involved. They may fail to recognize the toothbrush or how to use it, or put shaving cream on the brush instead of toothpaste. Some people drink mouthwash instead of swishing and spitting.

Getting the person to the dentist for care can be another challenge. Some people grow resistant to doctors, especially a person they see only once or twice a year. They may have trouble understanding what's being done to them or why it's important.

TRY this:

- Brush together. Sometimes copying a basic task is the easiest way to get it done (and you don't have to make a big deal about reminding). Obviously, this is easier for couples than, say, a parent and child.

- Set the brush, already loaded with toothpaste, on the sink when he goes to clean up. The visual prompt may lead to the task getting done.

- If he needs more help, break your verbal prompts into small steps: Pick up the brush. Put it in your mouth. Now brush it against the top teeth, and so on.

- Although brushing teeth after meals is ideal, this can be taxing. You might have better luck doing so in the mornings or whenever he's in a good mood. Waiting until evening, when he's tired, can make things harder.

- If he begins having trouble identifying personal-care items, consider removing things that might be swallowed or misused. Mouthwash is a common example.

- The right tools can help: Choose a soft brush. A thick handle is easier for many people to hold. Look for brushes designed for children that lack the cartoon characters or other juvenile elements. Some people prefer an electric toothbrush.

Tip: **"My dentist recommended a toothpaste containing fluoride to help keep cavities away because we have well water."— J.K.**

- Put dental care on your list of doctor visits. Make sure the dentist and hygienist are aware of the dementia before they treat. For troublesome cases, you might want to consider a dentist who specializes in dementia patients; it's a small but growing specialty. (To find one, search on "Alzheimer's" and "dentist" and your zip code or town.)

o o o

Grooming Trouble (Hairstyling, Make-Up, and Shaving)

Frank was never one to pay attention to his wife's make-up. All he knew is that Jackie always looked nice. She was a woman who liked to "pretty-up" for him, as he called it. True, her lipstick started to miss her lips a little bit, but he let it go. It made her happy to paint her face.

It rankled when his daughter pulled him aside to say, "Dad! Mom's starting to look like a clown! You can't let her go out like that!"

WHY it happens:

Personal grooming becomes a challenge for many reasons.

Someone may:

- Skip one or more grooming tasks out of forgetfulness

- Become unable to manage the complicated steps involved

- No longer identify the tools involved (comb, razor, lipstick) and how they're used

Minor grooming mistakes — where someone just looks "off" — are a common early sign of cognitive problems. When awareness is still good in the disease's early stage, she may know something's not right or be dissatisfied when grooming no longer comes out the way she'd like. She may redouble her efforts (sometimes making things worse) or begin to avoid them entirely.

TRY this:

Makeup:

- Avoid embarrassing the person with outright criticism. Aim to correct only in the mildest, most respectful terms, the way you might discreetly point out that someone has spinach in her teeth, for example.

- Consider shopping together or presenting lighter shades of lipstick that are more forgiving of errors in application, or a new gloss "that will make your lips feel soft."

- Casually offer help: "Here, maybe I can try that?" Or, "Want another pair of hands?"

- If certain kinds of makeup are really becoming a problem, you might "lose" them and see if they're missed.

- If makeup is being applied too heavily, she may not know when to quit. Narrowing the products can help.

Hair:

- Acknowledge efforts: "Your hair looks so nice today." Pat a stray piece into place while you say it, if needed.

- Let the stylist or barber know she has dementia when you book an appointment, to allow for extra time.

- Go short. Shorter cuts mean there's less to mess. A man might do well with short, cropped hair, especially if he once favored this look.

- Move away from an elaborate women's hairstyle, which is hard to maintain. As time goes on, it will also be harder to make regular appointments. Ask the stylist to "accidentally" cut hair extra-short, so you can go longer between trimmings. Exception: If a woman has a long tradition of a weekly salon visit, she may get pleasure in continuing. But don't keep it up for her out of loyalty once she no longer seems interested.

- Ask the stylist to shampoo hair first. A professional cleaning and conditioning will feel good and reinforce your efforts.

- Skip hair products (spray, gel, pomade, dye). Fewer steps make it easier. If you stop providing them — "Gee Dad, you're out" — eventually he'll forget them.

Shaving

- Prep the razor and lotion and give simple prompts at each step.

- Try an electric razor — it's less likely to nick. Some caregivers report fewer nicks (and fewer steps) with manual razors that have soap built into the cartridge.

Tip: **"My husband usually misses the whiskers on his neck. I make a joke and say, 'Oh, thanks, I see you left a little for me to do for you." — Amy**

- Encourage a man with dementia to quit shaving and grow a beard. Compliment his rugged good looks.

To help you cope:

- Know that grooming deficits can be hard on caregivers because they're a visual reminder that all's not really well with a loved one. Even when we tell ourselves that appearances shouldn't matter in the big scheme of things, it can tug at the heart a little.

Tip: **"It sounds corny, but a smile on Momma's face makes her look pretty to me, so that cancels out the goofy hair and the drawn-on crooked eyebrows. Now that's what I aim for, to get her to smile." — C.D.**

o o o

EATING PROBLEMS

Doesn't Eat, Won't Eat

Every afternoon, Gloria dropped off a hot meal for her father, who lived five minutes away. She also made sure his cupboards were stocked with cereal, fresh milk, and sandwich fixings for other meals. He'd never been much of a cook, and since her mother died, she wanted to be sure he ate well.

Lately she'd found the portions untouched. "Pops! Didn't you like the supper?" she'd ask, noticing lots of leftovers from the portions she'd bring him.

The time he ignored the lasagna was the last straw. "Your favorite! Aren't you feeling well?" That's when she began to look more closely into the refrigerator and cupboards. More often than not, she found the milk spoiled, the sandwich meat unopened. He ate heartily at her house but not in his own.

WHY it happens:

Not eating is a common problem that can have many different causes.

- *Cognitive challenges.* Someone who lives alone may find it too difficult to prepare food or even to deal with the sequence of steps involved with realizing it's time for a meal and heating up food that's been prepared in advance. — even though he's hungry.

- *Sensory changes.* People with Alzheimer's often have an impaired sense of smell. Aging generally can alter the senses of smell and taste, affecting appetite.

- *Not recognizing hunger.* People with dementia lose touch with bodily functions and what they mean.

- *Inactivity.* People who don't move around much eat less.

- *A physical problem.* Don't overlook causes unrelated to dementia, including a sore mouth, an upset stomach or other illness, a reaction to a new medication, or a problem with the fit of dentures, for example.

- *End-stage disease.* At the end of life, the body's systems start to shut down and loss of appetite is a natural part of this process. He'll often have great difficulty swallowing at this point, as well.

TRY this:

- Use clues about the situation to help pinpoint a cause. Is he losing weight? Is this a sudden change? Are there other signs of illness? Does it happen occasionally (finicky at certain meals) or at most meals? Does he have fairly late-stage dementia? Your exact approach will depend on the likely cause or causes.

- If you're at all concerned about weight loss or other physical factors, check in with a doctor.

- Reassess how he's getting food. Is someone available to prepare and serve every meal, or has he been doing some of this on his own? Is he's preparing meals on his own, is he struggling with this responsibility? It's possible more help is now needed. Look into Meals on Wheels or other local agencies that can deliver a daily hot meal.

- Be sure physical activity is also part of the daily routine, as much as is possible for the person's abilities.

- Tilt toward high-caloric, nutrition-dense foods for a birdlike eater. Good choices include dishes made with cheese, butter, nut butter, and whole milk. Casseroles (especially mad with recipes from older cookbooks) are often heavy on some of these ingredients. Shakes and smoothies made with fruit and whole milk yogurt, whole milk ice cream, or whole milk are also good.

- Try strongly flavored foods. Because taste buds dull for many people as they age, using more herbs, onion, garlic, or other seasonings may make food more appealing.

- Talk to the doctor about nutrition supplements that add

calories, such as Ensure or Boost. Note: These are different from so-called "medical foods," such as Axona, a controversial prescription-only nutrition supplement for Alzheimer's disease that provides the brain ketones for energy, rather than glucose. Axona is FDA-approved but not recommended by the Alzheimer's Association (which endorses no medical foods).

- Offer snacks throughout the day, such as high-calorie energy bars, oatmeal cookies, yogurt. Some people who tend to avoid big meals will willingly take a few bites if offered.

- Never force-feed, which is traumatic (no matter how good your intentions) and can be counterproductive.

What About Feeding Tubes?

Don't assume that a feeding tube is the most humane option when someone with late-stage disease shows little interest in eating. There's been a strong movement away from this method of treating people with advanced Alzheimer's disease. Caregivers tend to have high expectations for this treatment, according to an *Archives of Internal Medicine* study — hopes that the study found are rarely met.

Research shows that for those with advanced dementia, feeding tubes don't increase weight, improve nutrition, or help prevent aspiration pneumonia. Surprisingly, they don't even extend life. Feeding tubes tend to cause diarrhea and discomfort, while distancing the person from human touch.

The Alzheimer's Association's official position: "It is ethically permissible to withhold nutrition and hydration artificially administered by vein or gastric tube when the person with Alzheimer's disease or dementia is in the end stages of the disease and is no longer able to receive food or water by mouth."

Consult with medical staff and hospice professionals if you face this very difficult juncture. Know that it tends to be much harder to get a feeding tube removed than to have it placed, due to policies and permissions, especially in the absence of an advance directive about life support.

The more compassionate alternative: hand feeding ice chips and any food that will be taken (called assisted oral feeding). Don't fear that your loved one is "starving to death" as this is not what's happening in this situation. The body is already shutting down by natural process. Without food or water, the body releases endorphins, a substance that blunts pain.

o o o

Forgets Having Eaten, Wants More

One hot summer day, I cubed a big bowl of watermelon for my dad. "Thank you!" he said, digging in as he watched his baseball game.

I returned to the kitchen to finish the dishes and cut up some more fruit for myself.

"For me?" Dad said, pleased, as I entered the family room.

I was confused but handed him the bowl, figuring he was still hungry. My mother shouted from across the room in exasperation. "You just ate some!" To me, she said, "He does this all the time, lately!"

Dad didn't seem to recognize that the empty bowl beside him had been his. Whether you walked in with a bowl of watermelon, ice cream, nuts, popcorn — and whether or not he'd just polished off his own bowl — when Dad saw a snack bowl walk into the room while he was watching sports, that was action he wanted a piece of. — P.S.S.

WHY it happens:

An eroding short-term memory makes it hard for someone with dementia to remember what just happened. Add to this an inability to read the body's signals, such as hunger or satiety. When my dad sat down to watch a ballgame, that was the trigger for him to want to eat. Boredom can add to a desire to find pleasure in food.

Someone who says, "I'm hungry" may also be expressing (without fully realizing it) a hunger of a different sort — for attention, for affection, for something to do.

TRY this:

- Sidestep arguments or logic. ("But you just ate!") Someone with Alzheimer's at this stage can't follow a rational argument.

- Within reason, go ahead and offer the requested food if

it's reasonably harmless. But tread more carefully with empty calories that can cause his mood to crash and spoil his appetite for meals.

- Offer a hug and a distracting conversation: "Oh, we're all out of that. But let's plan the perfect dinner and I'll shop later. What would it be? What would be the first course?"

- Try breaking up the meal. Serve half now, half later. Or serve eggs and toast at breakfast, followed by fruit and yogurt for successive snacks.

- Offer a snack "to tide you over until it's ready." Something light might avoid an argument and make someone forget about wanting another full meal.

- Involve him in a busy activity after a meal to distract him, especially one involving the hands.

o o o

Gets Distracted During Meals

Elena usually comes to the table in a docile, agreeable way. But getting her to eat the meal can be vexing to her daughter, Maria. Elena goes through the right motions at the start — she puts her napkin in her lap, says a blessing, picks up her fork, and says, every time, "Why this looks delicious, dear."

But somewhere after the first forkful, Elena seems to forget why she's there. Her bites seem to slow down, and her attention wanders. As Maria's family talks about the day and gobbles down the meal, Elena often simply shuts down.

"Mama, eat!" Maria says every few minutes. Elena smiles, takes a bite...and then stops again.

WHY it happens:

The sheer number of steps involved with eating — recognizing hunger, connecting it to the food before you, following the steps involved in choosing to pick up a fork and fill it with food, and bring it to your mouth — can challenge someone with dementia. At every step of the way, competing interests, such as background noise, a decorative bowl of wax fruit on the table, or simply too many choices on the plate, can slow the process.

Some people will enter a stage of playing with their food. They simply forget what the food is or what should be done with it.

A frustratingly slow, indifferent eater isn't purposely annoying you. She can't help it.

TRY this:

- Help her focus on the meal at hand: Remove clutter from the table: papers, books, knick-knacks, centerpiece, napkin holders, salt and pepper shakers.

- Turn off the TV and turn the radio on or off. Soft music may help set a positive mood or be too distracting; experiment.

- Highlight the plate and cup by placing them on a contrasting solid placement (for example, a white plate on a black mat). A study in *Clinical Nutrition* found that people with Alzheimer's eat and drink more when using high-contrast tableware.

- Avoid patterns in dishes or table coverings. Solids are better because patterns can disorient or distract. Solid cups are less distracting than glass ones, through which liquid and distortion can se seen.

- Use the minimal number of utensils. If only a fork is needed, don't set out the full complement of knives and spoons. Skip the salad fork — just one utensil for the whole meal is fine. Metal is safer than plastic, which can be bitten off and swallowed without her realizing it.

- Put just one or two foods on the plate at a time, in small, manageable servings. (You can always add more after it's eaten.) A plateful of different choices may overwhelm.

- Make sure foods are the right temperature. If they're too hot, she may grow uninterested while waiting for something to cool.

- Especially with someone who stops eating or plays with food, offer calm, casual prompts through the meal to someone who needs this help (usually in later stages of the disease): "Pick up your fork...scoop the potatoes....take a bite...now swallow...isn't it good?" Better to encourage her to do it herself than to do it for her if she's physically capable of the mechanics.

- Use positive reinforcement before and during the meal so that good feelings are linked to the sight of the table. Talk about the delicious meal you're about to have, how good it smells.

- Avoid rushing through meals. Also avoid eating courses in unison so that everyone has to wait for the last person to finish. Put all the food out at once. If kids eat fast and finish early, excuse them rather than having them fidget and add tension.

To help you cope:

- Separate food from love in your mind. That's difficult for most of us, having been raised from childhood to find pleasure or reward in a cookie or to bask in pride when guests praise our dishes. Your friend or family member with Alzheimer's may still enjoy food, and yours in particular, but the disease makes it impossible for her to express this through words or deeds.

o o o

Messy Eating

I winced as Dad bit into the hot dog. Sure enough, big droplets of ketchup and mustard landed on his clean chinos. His napkin had already fluttered from his lap. Crumbs from the bun floated down next, landing in the sticky liquids. As usual, he seemed not to notice.

Half of every handful of potato chips made it into his mouth. The rest smashed against his cheek and crumbled to his lap. Too late, I replaced the napkin. I dabbed a ketchup blot from his lips. When he lifted a can of soda, I knew before it happened that at least some of the cola would dribble across his shirt.

Overall, the picnic was a success — Dad ate a full meal, he enjoyed listening to the live band and watching the grandchildren race around. But my sister's kindergartener went home cleaner than Grandpa did. — P.S.S.

WHY it happens:

Cognitive and physical changes combine to make it difficult to eat neatly. Some people lose some fine-motor control (over hands, utensils) and hand-eye coordination, either due to the dementia or another condition. At the same time, they tend to become less attentive to what they're doing or where the stray food bits are going. They may be oblivious about mess, both during the meal and after.

TRY this:

- Lower your expectations and look the other way as much as you can. Spills can be mopped. Clothes can be washed.

- Make sure the distance from chair to table is snug. Some chairs have heavy arms that don't fit under the table, so food must travel a little farther to get to the mouth.

- Unobtrusively place a napkin in the person's lap before serving food, if he no longer does this himself. It might not stay there, but it's a start.

- Cut up foods before serving them in manageable, bite-sized pieces. It can feel infantilizing to have the food on your plate cut for you, so either cut all the food before placing it in the serving dish or plate the food before you bring it to the table.

- To ease cleanup, try a vinyl tablecloth, which is easily wiped clean, or paper placemats that can be thrown away.

- Serve fewer messy foods, such as sauces and condiments (mustard, ketchup, mayo). Pre-season food before bringing it to the table.

- Switch to a "spork" — a combination spoon and fork — if manipulating utensils is difficult. (They're sold in camping stores or online.) Spoons are generally easier than forks, and anything with a thick handle is easier to grip.

- Try serving food in a bowl instead of a plate. Bowls better contain mess. Look for shallow, rimmed pasta dishes, which seem plate-like.

- Serve finger foods that eliminate the need to use a utensil. Examples: fried chicken, chicken strips, pizza cut into bite-sized squares, fish sticks, finger sandwiches, and unadorned vegetables such as green beans, diced squash, or roasted cubes of potato. Cook eggs omelet-style firm and cut them into strips or squares that can be picked up.

- At first, offer the finger-food meals to everyone at the table, so the person with dementia feels less singled out. Later, he may not notice.

- Serve soup in a mug that can be sipped, rather than a bowl. Let it cool a bit.

- You can also serve liquids in a lidded cup with a spout (available in hospital-supply stores). If you use a regular cup, pour it about a third full. Refill as needed.

- Find the most solid dishes you can, such as heavy ironstone, rather than fine china or thin melamine. Dishes with heft will be less likely to slip around.

- Choose heavy plastic cups over glass ones if grip is a problem. Solid colors are better than transparent glass, which can be disorienting to look through, adding to spills.

- If you point out a mistake (mustard smeared on the cheek, for example), do it in a casual way: "Oh that mustard got on you, too. Here, let me get it."

- Someone in the later stages might consent to wearing a smock apron during meals.

o o o

Won't Drink Enough Liquids

Emma had broken her wrist in a nighttime fall while still in her early 60s. Ever since, she'd been careful not to drink much in the evenings, so she wouldn't have to get up to go to the bathroom. As she got older and her bladder weakened, she'd begun avoiding liquids in the afternoons, too.

As her dementia progressed, Emma forgot many things. But the habit of not drinking liquids seemed to intensify. She refused anything to drink at any time of day. Her exasperated sister, Mary, was able to get her to take just a few sips with her pills but little more.

WHY it happens:

People with Alzheimer's may not get enough liquids for a variety of reasons:

- Often they lose the ability to "read" the sensation of thirst. And adults tend to feel less thirst generally as they age.

- Or they may be thirsty but not express it.

- They may simply forget to take sips along with meals or snacks during the day.

- They may avoid drinking, as Emma does, because they want to avoid the effects of liquids — having to get up to use the bathroom or difficulty in undressing and getting there in time. Some people want to avoid using the bathroom in public and will avoid drinking if they have to go to a doctor appointment or somewhere else.

The key risk to not drinking enough liquid is dehydration. It's a real risk among older adults with dementia, especially when the weather is warm or when taking medications that are dehydrating. This is another good reason to get familiar with the effects of drugs that the person in your care takes regularly.

TRY this:

- Offer liquids throughout the day; don't wait for her to ask. Aim for 6-8 total cups of fluid a day.

- Don't just hand over a glass; stand by and make sure the drink is actually sipped.

- Issue mild reminders during the meal: "Have a sip of water, Sis . . . try the iced tea."

- Vary the types of beverages offered: water, iced tea, juice, milk, hot chocolate, cider. Even coffee and soda are okay in moderation (about a cup a day) if your loved one prefers them. The latest thinking is that a cup or two a day doesn't pose a diuretic effect that would lead to dehydration. For someone not consuming enough liquids, liquids in any form are probably beneficial.

- Do, however, curb caffeinated beverages if fear of getting to the bathroom on time is an issue, since caffeinated drinks can cause frequent urination.

- Leave athletic water bottles around the house or carry them around during the day. Many older adults aren't in the habit of drinking this way, though, so if it doesn't work, don't press the point.

- Serve liquidy foods to make up some of the total. Fruit contains a lot of water, especially watermelon, melons like cantaloupe or honeydew, grapes, and citrus. Soup or broth is another option.

- For a liquid refusenik, invoke the doctor: "He wants you to drink this." Or, "He says this much is okay."

- For someone worried about getting to the bathroom on time, don't wait for her to need to go. Make the suggestion 20 to 30 minutes after drinking something. Make sure clothes are easy-on, easy-off, such as pants with elastic waistbands and no challenging belts.

- Be sure you know the symptoms of dehydration: increased confusion or lethargy, complaints of headache, dry skin or mouth, feeling warm to the touch. Call the doctor, who may recommend a rehydration solution (such as Pedialyte). If you can't rehydrate the person by getting her to take liquids and you don't see a change in symptoms, she may need IV (intravenous) hydration.

Know that diarrhea and vomiting increase the risk of dehydration, so monitor her especially closely when she's ill, and notify the doctor if you suspect dehydration.

o o o

HEALTH PROBLEMS

Confusion That Worsens Suddenly (Delirium)

Maria had to be hospitalized overnight when she'd begun to complain about chest pain, and family members were concerned an old replacement valve was no longer working well. Her daughter Aurelia stayed with her, catnapping on an easy chair next to the bed. A little after midnight, Maria awakened asking where her husband, Luis, was. Luis had died almost eight years earlier. At first Aurelia wasn't too concerned. Her mom sometimes forgot he'd died, and often mixed up lots of other dates and facts as her Alzheimer's had worsened.

But then Maria began to babble in Spanish. Though fluent, Aurelia could nevertheless make out only bits and pieces because her mother was talking so fast and yet in fragments. Maria seemed to be talking about flying over fields of corn looking for Luis. She heard her comment how pretty the sunshine was, how much she enjoyed flying, and how they had to get home before her father caught them.

"Then she started to grow more agitated, clutching at the bed sheets and calling everybody's name: Luis! Papa! Aurelia! All of us mixed together. It almost sounded like a dream, but she was wide awake," Aurelia says. "And she would not respond to me or focus on me.

"It was very scary and went on for some time."

Aurelia was sure that just being in the hospital had caused her mom's Alzheimer's to worsen. Then she found out that her mother had developed a urinary tract infection, quite separate from the heart issue. After a week on antibiotics, Maria seemed to return to the way she was before the hospitalization.

WHY it happens:

Delirium — a reversible state of acute mental confusion — is usually caused by a stress that affects the whole body. This stress could be any number of things:

- a known or new infection (like pneumonia, UTI, or a skin infection)

- low oxygen level (brought on by heart attack or a lung exacerbation from COPD)

- a medication reaction

- sleep deprivation

- pain

- dehydration

- acute emotional stress, including depression or a psychiatric condition.

One 2013 study found that more than half of all people with dementia who are hospitalized will experience delirium. The risk is also higher when someone in the hospital is dehydrated, an alcoholic, or undergoing anesthesia.

Delirium isn't a disease; it's a syndrome of changes caused by an underlying problem. As brain function is scrambled due to the delirium, it causes behaviors that are sometimes your only clue to a life-threatening illness. That's why it's important for a family caregiver to be able to recognize it. Doctors and nurses often miss it because they don't know your loved one as well as you do — and often attribute what they're seeing to the fact that the person has dementia.

The signs of delirium vary from person to person. There's no single way someone acts delirious. So trust your intuition. When a caregiver senses something's "off" about a loved one's behavior or functioning, there's often a very real reason for it.

Here are the most common signs of delirium in someone with dementia:

- **A sudden turn for the worse in the usual state of mental impairment** The change usually happens over a period of hours but sometimes comes on more gradually (over days). Look for a change in what's normal for your loved one (whatever the current, demented normal is).

- **Fluctuating confusion** A tricky aspect of delirium is that the mental changes in awareness and orientation come and go. The person may alternate between seeming fine at moments and seeming much more confused than usual at other times. Your loved one may already (due to the dementia) have good days and bad days, or good and bad times of day. So how can you identify changes associated with delirium? The problem is similar to that of parents trying to assess whether a child is truly sick versus just having a fussy day. Look for patterns in a typical day — for example, many people with dementia ordinarily have better mornings than late afternoons. In that case, extra confusion that appears in the morning might be a red flag.

- **Difficulty paying attention** The person has trouble focusing (on conversation, on anything).

- **Agitation, being more revved up than usual** This can range from a surge in nervous energy to increased combativeness or anger. Someone who's usually mild-mannered may behave aggressively.

- **Acting much quieter or drowsier** Although "being delirious" tends to call up images of raving madness, in many people delirium manifests as becoming quieter and more spaced out. This is called *hypoactive delirium* and is just as dangerous.

- **Hallucinations/delusions** The person doesn't act like his or her usual self. He or she may see or hear things that aren't real, make false accusations, or otherwise not be grounded in reality. In someone with dementia who already has been having hallucinations or delusions, they may be more frequent or troubling.

Once you notice the first possible signs of delirium, pay even closer attention to possible other changes over the next hours and days. And be prepared to act quickly if you do see signs.

TRY this:

After you notice signs of delirium:

- Start with a medical evaluation, quickly. If you're at home, call 911 or go to the emergency room if you notice signs of delirium and there's also been a serious fall, a head injury or broken bone, or the person is having trouble staying conscious or breathing. If these crisis signs don't apply, it's still a good idea to get an urgent-care appointment, at the person's primary care provider if you can. If you're already in a hospital, alert staff. Let them know you suspect delirium and why.

  Fast action matters because, while there's no drug that treats delirium, the treatment is usually a matter of identifying and treating the underlying cause. Once this happens, the delirium usually improves in a matter of hours or days (although in elderly adults it can take weeks or even months to get back to their best mental selves. Delirium also predisposes a person with dementia to acceleration of memory loss, another reason a quick response, and treatment, is important.

- Don't count on hospital staff to notice delirium. It can be hard to identify in someone who "normally" has confusion and memory loss. Trust your instincts. You know your loved one's normal status better than anyone. Be persistent about pointing out what seems different about your loved one so it doesn't get written off as "but she has dementia." You'd be surprised how often even doctors and nurses fail to recognize delirium in patients, especially in those who already have Alzheimer's or other forms of dementia.

- Stay with the person during an evaluation. You have to be there to express what's typical and answer any questions.

- Bring all medications to an evaluation. That includes prescriptions, over-the-counter drugs for pain, colds, and allergies, and nutritional supplements. These are a common cause or contributor to delirium. Don't forget medications that were started and stopped for any reason or that recently ran out or ended.

- Pay attention to the work-up for delirium. A good doctor will investigate possible underlying causes by doing a physical exam (looking for fever and other signs of infection, for example, and taking vital signs and possibly ordering blood or urine tests). Pain will also be assessed, such as following a fall or from constipation. People with Alzheimer's often fail to report their pain, so the doctor can't rely the patient's word on this, in this case. Finally, the work-up should include a medications review.

To prevent delirium:

- Pay attention to keeping the person hydrated. Even healthy older adults tend to drink less liquid than they should. Older adults with dementia can simply forget and lose the ability to read their body's signals for thirst. This can worsen in hot weather or when someone's feeling under the weather. In the study that showed half of all hospitalized dementia patients experience delirium, one third of these patients were found to be dehydrated on admittance (though that wasn't the reason for the hospitalization).

- If your loved one must ever be hospitalized, arrange for someone to stay with her throughout the stay, 24/7. Someone with any degree of cognitive impairment is unable to keep track of what doctors say and do, much less speak up for herself about her symptoms and needs. Moreover, a hospital can be a distressing and disorienting place for someone with Alzheimer's. Your steady, familiar presence can go a long way to reducing stress. You'll also be able to identify signs of delirium (as Aurelia noticed with her mother) and can alert hospital staff.

- If you have the option, look for a hospital with an acute-care-for-elders (ACE) unit, a growing option.

- In the hospital, make sure that glasses, hearing aids, and other assistive devices needed by the patient are handy. They're often taken off for sleep or a procedure, and in the hospital hubbub, not returned — contributing to disorientation. You know what your loved one uses; the night nurse doesn't. Provide extra orienting reminders: "You're in the hospital to have your heart checked." Say it over and over. Don't be shy about asking medical staff what can be done to ensure that the patient gets enough to drink (to avoid dehydration) and gets enough sleep (especially at night, when checks and medication dispensing can disorient someone with Alzheimer's).

By some estimates, nearly half of delirium cases in hospitals can be eliminated through steps like these.

o o o

Constipation

Gerald didn't seem like himself. He moaned a lot. But he couldn't exactly say what was wrong. His wife, Gloria, felt his forehead — no fever. She put her hands on his arms and legs, but he didn't seem to have any tender spots. He didn't flinch when she touched his back and knees, places where his arthritis had always been most severe. But he wouldn't stop moaning.

Then he didn't even want to eat. Alarmed, she took him to the doctor.

Gerald's arthritis is severe enough that he starting taking a prescription pain reliever several months ago. It seems to have helped the pain — but has had an often-unrecognized side effect. It causes constipation.

WHY it happens:

Constipation is defined as having pain or difficulty emptying the bowels, or straining for several minutes, usually due to hard stool. As a rule of thumb, going three days without a bowel movement (BM) is a flag for constipation. But in general, the goal is to have a comfortable BM every one to two days.

Alzheimer's isn't normally a cause (constipation can happen to anyone), but people with Alzheimer's do have a few added strikes against them:

- People with cognitive impairment tend to lose the ability to read their body's signals. Unable to know when they're hungry or thirsty, they're at higher risk of dehydration, which can cause constipation. Also they may not be aware when they need to use the bathroom.

- They have a hard time articulating pain of impacted BMs.

- They often become less active and sit more, raising the risk.

- They may be prescribed anticholinergics (including Benadryl and/or narcotic pain relievers), which raise the risk.

229

- People with non-Alzheimer's dementias such as Parkinson's or Lewy Body can develop constipation when the nerves of the digestive system are affected.

- The incidence of constipation rises with age, as does dementia.

Untreated, constipation can darken mood and escalate behavior problems. Chronic constipation can also lead to fecal impaction, in which feces stuck in the bowels causes other health problems. People who use laxatives for a long time are at added risk of this.

"Constipation is considered a less-than-glamorous topic by doctors, but proper treatment can make a world of difference to an older patient," says San Francisco geriatrician Leslie Kernisan.

TRY this:

To prevent constipation problems:

- In general, offer plenty of liquids. Remember, it doesn't have to be water. Also good: soup, pulpy orange juice, thin hot cereal (such as diluted Cream of Wheat), frozen fruit bars, lemonade.

- Serve a diet that includes plant foods and whole-grain fiber. Realize, though, that certain medications will create a tendency to constipation separate from a healthy diet.

- Consider this yet another reason for your loved one to walk around and have other physical activity each day.

- Watch for facial grimaces, listen for grunting or other signs of pain when your loved one uses the toilet. You might catch on early to a case of constipation, so it can be treated.

- Don't obsess over BMs (not everyone goes every day). But to prevent a repeat episode, it can help to track toileting habits so you have a sense when it's been awhile and notice other symptoms (such as grimacing or pain).

230

To treat constipation:

- Talk to the doctor about the best option to get things moving in the individual's case. There are many options, and some can be bought at your local drugstore, but they each have different pros and cons. Be sure to mention to the doctor whether you're dealing with acute or chronic constipation. Acute constipation requires something to get the person unplugged. Most older adults are chronically a bit constipated and need to figure out what kind of regimen will keep them regular.

- Ask about the options. Dr. Kernisan notes that the four main types of laxatives used for constipation are:

1. Osmotic agents (laxatives with non-absorbable sugars) to draw water into the bowel. This makes stool softer. Prune juice is one choice. The over-the-counter drug MiraLax is another. There are also prescription alternatives.

2. Stimulating agents to act directly on the colon stimulate the muscles. The OTC agent senna is one choice, or a suppository may be prescribed.

3. Softening agents to make the stool softer and more slippery. The best known and most prescribed is Colace, but it's not as effective as the other choices.

4. Fiber "bulking agents" to bulk up the stool in order to get the colon working right. The OTC powder Metamucil is a popular example. Fiber has to be taken with a lot of water so it doesn't stop things up. And it can cause gas and bloating — so it's not a good choice for everyone.

Sometimes a combination of these is recommended. Dr. Kernisan also emphasizes that most older adults take some laxative every day and that it shouldn't be cause for concern. It's generally safe, and the benefits greatly outweigh the small theoretical risk, she says.

Be wary of lowering pain medication to avoid or lessen constipation. In general, older adults tend to receive too little pain med, not too much. It's better for the patient to treat the symptom of constipation than to try to eliminate it by cutting out the pain drug causing it, Kernisan cautions.

o o o

Incontinence and Adult Diapers *

My grandmother, then in her early 90s and fairly deep in her dementia, was living with my cousin when she began to have "accidents." Not that she drew any attention to them, at least not with her words. Instead she'd remove the wet underpants and carefully set them out to dry...on the radiator. "You'd walk in the front door and — whew! Instant nursing home smell," my cousin recalls.

Once (when nobody was home) she got a large cooking pot from the kitchen, used it as a makeshift commode — and replaced it on its shelf, without a word. — P.S.S.

(* NOTE: It's best to avoid using the word diapers when talking to your loved one because it's demeaning and outdated. I've used it here only because this is how people often search for information about incontinence and personal-care products.)

WHY it happens:

Incontinence — loss of bladder or bowel control — can be part of the progression of Alzheimer's and is also a result of other problems someone with Alzheimer's might be having. Any accidents can be dicey to discuss with a loved one, given the privacy and embarrassment surrounding the issue. An added challenge is that by the time dementia-related accidents begin, the person is usually deep into the disease and lacks the insight and logic to respond in a straightforward way.

Someone with Alzheimer's who starts having accidents might hide them, as in my Gram's case. Or she may react obliviously, every time. My dad used to try to outsmart the problem by unzipping right in the hallway, all the better to make it to the commode on time (with mixed results). Those who are delusional might try to blame other people — "He threw water on my bed."

Non-Alzheimer's causes, many of which are treatable, can include:

- Chronic urinary issues due to overactive bladder, prostate issues (men), and/or pelvic muscle relaxation (women)

- Urinary tract infections

- Medication reactions

- Certain food or drink triggers (such as colas and caffeine).

TRY this:

- Start by recognizing that "job one" isn't to get the person into wearing incontinence products. It's to get a doctor to rule out any possible medical problems, especially if the incontinence is new or getting worse. It's always better to address the situation this way rather than avoid it, hoping it will go away. Many causes for incontinence are treatable, and some cases will go away entirely. You don't have to make a big deal about it as the purpose of a doctor visit if you're worried your loved one might be embarrassed. Make an appointment on the pretext of something else — say, a flu shot or a medication check — and alert the staff in advance.

- A bonus with starting with the doctor is that he or she can "prescribe" the incontinence products, so you have a neutral third party recommending them, and you don't have to play the bad guy.

- Have empathy — even though dealing with this problem can be really, really annoying, especially when it happens for the second or third time in the middle of the night. Someone with dementia is not "doing it on purpose" or "doing it to get back at you." Loss of bladder control means just that — she can't control it.

- Realize that early in dementia, you're apt to be as uncomfortable talking about the subject as the incontinent person is. (Later, it's common to encounter less resistance — but not always.) Being matter of fact and approaching it as a health issue, not a personal one, works best. Humor can help for some: "Well, you finally have something in common with those famous old TV stars on the commercials!"

- Keep repeating what the "doctor says." The person with dementia isn't going to remember and needs to be reminded of new behaviors. It often helps to invoke the doctor — that neutral third party who can take the heat off of you as the "bad guy."

- Show you're on her side: "I know you hate this, but the doctor thinks we can find out why this is happening." "I know it's annoying for you, but the doctor says if we do x and y...." No one likes wetting herself, but everyone tends to feel relieved about the prospect of taking action.

- Consider a wardrobe change. Sometimes people fall into the habit of wearing the sorts of clothes they've always worn, but these outlive their usefulness when the goal is getting to the bathroom quickly. Men might be able to skip wearing a belt, for example, or switch to pants with a large zipper. (No button flies or overalls!) Both genders can switch to pull-down sweatpants or elastic-waist pants. Women with incontinence do better without stockings.

- Make the bathroom easy to use. Among the improvements caregivers report success with: A taller-than-normal commode (easier to sit down on); grab bars near the toilet; a toilet seat in a contrasting color to the commode (for example, a dark seat in an all-white bathroom will aid someone with depth-perception).

- Consider a bedside commode. Trips to the bathroom in the dark and night can be slower than usual. Be sure there isn't a wastebasket nearby that might be mistaken for a commode.

- Look for cues she needs to go. These might be obvious (pulling at pants, wiggling) or more subtle (a certain facial expression or increasing agitation, for example).

- Pay attention to whether the person starts to use special, mixed-up language to refer to the need to use the toilet or to having had an accident. It's typical for someone with dementia to refer to rain or showers, for example.

- Keep a toileting schedule for a while to track when your she needs to use the toilet or has accidents. You'll probably be able to find a pattern and can lead her to the bathroom in advance.

- Offer verbal reminders. Because you can't rely on her body to signal when she needs to use the bathroom, it helps for you to say so: "It's a long drive; let's go to the bathroom before we go." "We're walking past the restroom, so let's go in."

- Look into incontinence products. You might be surprised by the range of options. There are products that resemble underwear, and come in different styles for men and women.

- If the person remains resistant to using incontinence products, try to emphasize the advantages: *We'll be able to stay out longer, you can go to your program without embarrassment, you'll feel more comfortable, the modern kind are so good nobody can even tell what they are.*

- Or point out how common they are. ("Why do you think they make so many of them?")

- Watch your language. Avoid using the word "diapers," which is demeaning, when talking about the products together. Better: *Briefs, panties, special pants, protective underwear* or just *new underpants.*

- Try to switch out the old underwear cold turkey, rather than making their use optional. Someone with dementia might have an easier time getting used to a change this way, when there's no visual reminder of old underthings.

Don't stop at undergarments. Ask the doctor about which

lotions, cleansers, and skin barriers would be best to protect your loved one's skin. People with bowel and bladder accidents are at a higher risk of bedsores, infections, and other skin problems.

Invest in waterproof sheets, bedcovers, and chair pads, too. Though not inexpensive, they can save you a lot of grief.

Be aware that someone with moderate dementia may not be able to identify when an incontinence garment is wet or full. You may need to double check, so she doesn't keep the same one on all day as if it were actual underwear.

Tip: **"If I say Mom's briefs are 'wet' she gets mad and says 'no they're not.' If I say they look 'heavy,' she'll change right away." — E.L.**

To help you cope:

- Avoid comparing your situation to others; you have to do what's best for you on this one. Allow that this is a problem that varies from situation to situation. For some caregivers, persistent incontinence ultimately becomes a "deal breaker" that necessitates a move out of a private home. Others find that the problem is manageable and don't mind so much. But how you experience it can depend on many factors, including the severity of the problem, whether you're encountering both bowel and bladder incontinence, what kind of help is available, the person's mobility, and your relative sizes (since help with toileting is a physical task).

o o o

Sleeps Too Little, Disturbed Sleep

"Oh no, not again." Rick looked at the clock: 3:15. It was the third time his mother-in-law had been up that night, rapping on their bedroom door. He rolled over and wrapped the pillow over his head.

Carol sighed, too. She couldn't go back to sleep, though. She knew her mother, Betty, would keep on knocking. An hour ago, she'd awakened their teenage son — and he usually slept through anything!

Sometimes Betty simply woke up and could be heard rummaging around in her room. If she left the room to use the bathroom, however, all bets were off. She'd travel from the bathroom to the kitchen, see nobody there, and proceed to wander through the house looking for them, until she came to Rick and Carol's locked bedroom door. And the knocking would begin.

At first, when this pattern started, Carol thought her mother needed help in the bathroom. Then she tried soothing her back to sleep with some warm milk and a gentle back rub. Some nights, this did the trick. Other nights, Carol would finally turn on the TV and let her mom fall asleep in front of it — which worked for a few precious hours at a stretch.

WHY it happens:

The effects of Alzheimer's on sleep aren't fully understood. Because sleep's control centers lie deep within the brain, the changes that occur there due to disease can in turn disrupt the natural rhythms that govern sleep. One common pattern: Oversleeping by day, or feeling drowsy during the day, and then feeling more wakeful at night. Alzheimer's medications can disrupt sleep in some patients.

What's all too well understood, however, is that disrupted sleep is one of the biggest problems many caregivers face. A loved one's sleep trouble becomes your sleep trouble, too.

Without enough sleep, someone with Alzheimer's becomes more irritable, confused, and prone to acting out with difficult behaviors. There's an association between lack of sleep and agitated behaviors. Caregivers, in turn, who function on too-little sleep can also experience fuzzy thinking, fatigue, changes in mood, weight gain, and more. There's growing evidence that lack of sleep is linked to chronic diseases such as high blood pressure, diabetes, heart disease, and depression. So it's a serious matter.

On top of the brain changes of dementia, it's possible that insomnia and restless sleeping are being caused by a factor other than Alzheimer's. These causes might include:

- Sleep apnea, in which someone stops breathing momentarily; it's linked to obesity. There's also a relationship to dementia, since people who have apnea seem to be more likely to develop Alzheimer's.

- An overactive bladder, causing night waking or incontinence.

- Restless legs syndrome — a tingling sensation creates a strong urge to keep moving your legs. One in 10 American adults have this, and the incidence increases with age.

- Depression. Sleep disruptions are a major sign of depression, which itself occurs more often in people who have dementia.

- Medication reactions. Beta blockers, for example, can cause insomnia, and diuretics can wake you up to relieve your bladder.

- Pain — whether from a known or unknown condition — can disrupt sleep.

- Age. Adults of all ages need about the same amount of sleep (7 to 8 hours). But sleep cycles change so that an older adult spends more time in light sleep, compared to deep sleep.

These common sleep problems are health threats for anyone. (You may experience some of them yourself.) When you also have dementia, however, it's harder to follow treatments or to self-calm and get back to sleep. The ensuing agitation and disruption then becomes an issue for the whole household.

Part of the reason the problem is so tough is that a combination of causes (brain changes, other physical causes, depression, medications, age) can all be in play at once.

TRY this:

- Start with trying to alter behavior or the environment. Both over-the-counter and prescription sleep medications have many side effects that can backfire, ranging from raising the risk of dangerous falls to increased mortality, so they're considered a last resort. What's more, studies don't show the effectiveness for the usual sleep aids such as Ambien for people with Alzheimer's. Some caregivers report success with the hormone melatonin, but clinical trials have shown no effect, perhaps because people with Alzheimer's have fewer melatonin receptors, according to a Johns Hopkins report.

- Stick to a predictable daily routine, in which the day begins and ends at about the same times. Daytime naps should also come at the same time and be about the same length each day.

- Review the daily routine:

- Does it include exposure to sunlight in the morning? Bright light, soon after waking, can help reset the body's inner clock and encourage sleep later.

- Is there time to get outside and get some exercise — even just walking around the house and yard? If you're already taking one walk a day, try taking two.

- Are naps kept to a minimum? Hours of napping midday, especially after lunch or dinner, will interfere with evening sleep.

- Are meals at about the same time each day? They're key

to a consistent routine.

- Is the evening wind-down calming? Dim the lighting when the sun goes down and keep activities after dinner to the quiet side (no loud TV!).

- Do you use the same sleep cues each night when it's time to turn in? Follow the same series of soothing events nightly. For example, shut all the shades, serve a small mug of warm cocoa, help her brush teeth and wash up, and play classical music softly in her room.

- In addition to getting bright morning light, keep the living area bright during the day. Open curtains, turn on lights on gloomy days, and get outside or seat your loved one near a window. Lots of light helps to regulate the body's natural circadian rhythm, and sends a message to your loved one that, "This is day; this is when we're up." Then in the evening, especially on the long days of summer, start to close curtains and dim the house as a prep for the message, "This is night; when we sleep."

- Reserve the bedroom for sleep, if you can. It can be hard, since in many homes space is precious and the bedroom of the older adult with dementia is set up as a refuge for sitting, watching TV, and so on. But if you can spare the space, linking the room to sleep-only sometimes helps.

- Follow "sleep hygiene" basics: Make sure the bedroom is on the cool side, with comfortable blankets for warmth. It's best if it's dark, although you need light to guide her to the bathroom; one solution is motion-sensor nightlights.

Tip: **"My wife is calmed by the humming sound of a fan. It's white noise that covers up street sounds. I run it even in winter, on low." — R.R.**

- Avoid laying out the next day's clothes at night when you're grappling with sleep issues. Do it after the person wakes up in the morning, to act as a visual cue to get up and get dressed.

- When she wakes up at night, avoid turning on bright lighting or the television; keep a consistent sense of difference between day and night.

- Don't feel you need to stay up until she falls back asleep if you're confident that she's safe. Offer a quiet activity, such as a book on tape or playing the same classical music she listens to before going to bed. (TV is often too stimulating for many people, who mistake the scenes on the screen for real events and get worked up over them.) Some caregivers have had success using a baby monitor to keep tabs on a wakeful person in another room; it might provide enough sound contact to reassure you that she's okay and let you fall back asleep without getting out of bed yourself.

- Pay attention to caffeine consumption. Many older adults have a big coffee habit. Caffeine not only peps you up, it's a diuretic that makes you need to go to the bathroom. Try to wean your loved one off coffee and caffeinated tea after midday if sleep is becoming an issue.

- Also beware of alcohol use, especially in the afternoon or evening. A "nightcap" can make someone fall asleep — and then awaken a short time later.

- Avoid all "nighttime medicines" (PM in the name) and antihistamines, which can worsen sleep.

- Consider hiring night help, if you can afford it, to protect your own sleep. If night-wakings are chronic, an aide who works the overnight shift can help your loved one with toileting and getting back to sleep.

- When behavioral strategies aren't working and your own health is in jeopardy, report persistent disrupted sleep to the doctor. (Several times a week is a good rule of thumb.) He or she can look for other underlying causes, such as depression. Have the doctor review all medications, as well. In some cases, a referral to a sleep specialist can help (for a problem such as apnea, for example), but the person should have experience dealing with dementia (a geriatrician is best). What works for someone without dementia may not apply in your loved one's case.

Your doctor may explore sleep aids. Antipsychotic meds are used in some extreme cases, but they don't generally work for insomnia, according to the American Psychiatric Association and American Geriatric Society's "Choosing Widely" campaigns about smart care practices.

Tip: **"My husband had more sleep problems when he took Aricept in the evening. We switched it to the morning on the doctor's advice, and the problem really improved." — S.B.**

To help you cope:

- Take sleep problems seriously. Don't just "suck it up" and consider chronic sleep deprivation to be part of the bargain of Alzheimer's care. Occasional mixed-up days and some rough nights are one thing. But when the disruptions are chronic and extreme, spending the time and money to resolve the issue is critical. The health risks to yourself are just too great and too well documented.

  It's absolutely worth it to bring in reinforcements: consulting a doctor, hiring night help. You may even want to hire an elder companion for an hour or so a day to give you time to nap.

- Explore whether a change in care situations is the best solution. When a sleep problem is really intractable (or in-home support isn't viable) it can be a message that it's time to explore an alternate care situation. Many caregivers resist their loved one moving from home, only to find that everyone's health improves on the move (some nursing homes even have nighttime activities to satisfy the mixed-up schedules of night owl residents) — leaving the caregiver better able to be an advocate, companion, and beloved figure to the person with

Alzheimer's. Every case is different, but sleep really brings home the adage, *never say never.*

o o o

Sleeps Too Much

Some days, Su seemed fine. She'd sit around the house and watch TV, pet her cats, or "look at" the paper. But other days, she didn't want to get out of bed. If coaxed up, she'd fall asleep on the sofa after breakfast and sleep all day. She'd doze right through lunch and dinner. Her husband, Warren, first worried that all that sleep would keep her up at night, but she'd continue to sleep at night, too.

Then he worried about that. Is it possible to sleep too much?

WHY it happens:

Sleep is controlled deep in the brain. It's not surprising, then, that disrupted sleep patterns are a common effect of the brain erosion of Alzheimer's.

Stage of disease matters. Some people with mild-stage dementia report feeling excessively tired, possibly from working so hard to stay "with it" and "on" all day. Moderate dementia is when the more wakeful sleep problems typically pick up. In end-stage Alzheimer's, it's normal for the person to sleep more and more as a natural part of the dying process. The body is slowly shutting down. (By this point, you'll see other signs of late-stage Alzheimer's, as well, possibly including difficulty swallowing, inability to talk or walk, not seeming to recognize close family, and so on. This doesn't mean the end is imminent — a person can continue in this state for many months, even years.)

Other possible causes (or additional causes):

- An underlying physical problem, such as an infection. Excessive lethargy can be a warning sign of delirium.

- A medication interaction or side effect.

- Depression. Disordered sleep is one of the key warning signs.

While sleeping too little or too erratically tends to cause more problems for caregivers, sleeping too much can also be problematic. The lack of a consistent schedule can, over time, make someone cranky and erratic. This can cause other behavior problems to increase. Or, over time, the person's day and night schedule can flip-flop.

In general, people think and feel better and have more energy when sleep is regular. Excessive daytime sleep can lead to disturbed behavior in the evening.

TRY this:

- Keep a log of sleep for a week or two. Include day and night sleep and any wakings for toileting or other reasons. That record can help you and the doctor figure out what might be going on.

- Mention excessive sleep to the doctor, especially if it's a recent change or if there are behavioral and mood changes, too. You want to make sure there isn't some other problem causing sleep changes, including a medication reaction.

- For someone who's fairly "with it" when awake, make sure that she gets regular exercise (walking counts) and time outdoors. Too much sleep can make people drowsy, but movement peps them up and makes them more likely to sleep normally.

o o o

Walking Trouble, Shuffling

One of the more distressing physical changes in my dad was the way he walked. Even deep in his retirement, through his 70s, he'd traipse a half mile to buy the daily newspaper rather than get home delivery. He resisted a golf cart longer than many of his buddies. But as his dementia took hold, his entire body seemed to turn more frail.

Going anywhere was an excruciating lesson in patience, as he slooooooowly maneuvered out of the car and began to walk. He was still mobile through the end of his life, but he seemed to have trouble picking up his feet and moving them along.

I didn't learn until later that he was doing the "Alzheimer's shuffle" — a common kind of impaired gait. — P.S.S.

WHY it happens:

A shuffling walk reflects the difficulty that the brain and body are having communicating. As the parietal lobe part of the brain, which governs motor skills, is affected, so is muscle coordination. He has trouble picking up his feet to walk and drags them a bit. You may also notice that he's unsteady and begins to stoop. Sometimes you see him concentrating harder on each step.

Although families don't often pick up on a slowing gait until the middle of Alzheimer's, some research indicates changes in walking may actually be one of the earlier symptoms. Gait changes can be seen even before memory changes. Movement involves the nervous system (sending messages throughout the body) as well as the heart and muscles. Some studies have revealed that people with cognitive impairment show more pronounced trouble walking when asked to do a thinking-skill task at the same time. As they divert focus to the cognitive task, their walking worsens. Slow walking speed is also associated with more cognitive decline.

A shuffle can be worsened by a fear of falling, due to changes in depth perception or orientation caused by Alzheimer's. The apprehension makes the person take more tentative steps. (Ironically, fear of falling is one of the risk factors for falling more.)

A medication reaction or other chronic diseases that add to overall frailty can also contribute to shaky walking. Medications that worsen balance include anticholinergics (found in overactive bladder drugs, PM painkillers, and some antidepressants), sedatives, some blood pressure meds, and opiate painkillers.

Falls are the real danger here. A quarter of those who fall and break a hip die within six months, and half can't return to a private home but must permanently relocate to a nursing facility.

Someone with vision problems, whether related to Alzheimer's or a pre-existing condition, is at added danger of falling.

TRY this:

- Make sure shoes fit well. Look for soles that offer some traction, neither too slick nor too rigid, such as canvas sneakers or sport sandals with secure back straps. Beware sport shoes with super-thick treads. These can actually contribute to falls because when the wearer can't lift his foot enough, they stick to the carpet. While laces are ideal for a snug fit, they can come undone and be tripping hazards and are hard for someone with poor flexibility and muscle-control issues to tie. Stick with Velcro straps. Ninety percent of all women wear shoes that are too small, says the American Association of Orthopedic Surgeons. Older adults tend to go by the size they've "always been" or don't realize how easy it now is to find wide-width shoes.

- Don't overlook safe slippers, since people with dementia often move around a lot at night. Slippers should have treads, too, and fasten securely to feet.

- Consider encouraging bare feet indoors. An Irish study in the journal *Age and Ageing* reported that frail older women who wore shoes fell more than those who went barefoot.

- Provide a cane, walking stick, or walker to boost support and, in turn, confidence. Of the three, walkers carry the lowest risk of falling — but they're often met with more resistance at first. (Medicare covers walkers.) Many people resist them because it makes them feel "old." Emphasize the advantages of a walking device — *you'll be able to walk better or farther, exercise will help you grow stronger, and you'll be less likely to fall and break a bone, which will really make you feel old.*

- When walking in stores, encourage a shuffling walker to push a shopping cart. It can provide just the right added support.

- Offer constant reminders to use the assistive device, since someone with Alzheimer's is likely to forget. Store it in view as a visual reminder.

- Lower the risk of accidental trips by getting rid of throw rugs, piles of paper, loose electric cords, and any other objects that clutter pathways. Pet toys are a surprising source of danger.

- Beware of two-toned rugs or other places where there's a contrast in floor color on one level. This can be perceived as a step, causing the person to jerk the leg up on a level surface. The very best floor coverings for someone with walking and perception problems: monotone, low-pile, wall-to-wall carpeting that extends seamlessly into hallways and other rooms.

- Offer extra support on steps and curbs. Changes in depth perception can make it easy to misjudge these distances, putting someone with dementia off balance.

Tip: "I painted the steps from the house down to the garage in alternating colors, red and white. Before, the concrete made them all look the same. The stripes are funky, but the contrast really helps my mother — and it helps me, too! — J.R.

- Mention any trouble walking to the doctor at the next checkup, especially if it's a recent change or if there's been a change in medications. It's always smart to rule out other causes or treat them.

- Ask about a referral to a physical therapist or occupational therapist. These experts won't be able to make the Alzheimer's shuffle go away, but they can evaluate balance and gait, and offer advice on how to best reduce the risk of falls, including showing how to use a walking assistive device.

- Make sure vision checks are up-to-date.

- Do what you can to keep the person moving, even if it's slow. Regular movement can reduce the risk of falls.

- Resist the urge to try to hurry the person along with your words. Saying, "Hurry!" Or, "We'll be late!" only adds stress and can tank your progress.

To help you cope:

- Allow more time to get places. You'll feel less maddened with impatience if you get in the habit of building in time for the slowed pace.

- Go a little Zen in your head: Take deep breaths and remind yourself that all that matters is this moment, and this next step, and the next.

o o o

"Alzheimer's is a family disease."

— Carol Burnett, actress and comic

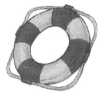

3 PERSONAL AND FAMILY STRESSORS

What helps when "everything else" undermines you

At one point, my brother Paul and sister-in-law Laura had three parents living with them. Only one had dementia (my dad), but the entire trio was north of age 75 and the myriad health issues between them — cancer, congestive heart failure, vertigo, to name a few — could fill a medical encyclopedia. Oh, and this cozy, crazy abode also housed six kids under age 13, three cats, and two dogs. (Luckily, my brother's a builder and kept remodeling his house accordingly.)

Not surprisingly, my sister-in-law, a.k.a. The Saint, soon developed terrible insomnia. She often couldn't eat. Some days, despite her mile-long to-do list, she couldn't get out of bed. Finally one night, her symptoms landed her in the E.R.

Diagnosis: Physically healthy but emotionally and mentally exhausted.

As part of her long road to learning to take care of herself as well as she took care of everyone else, we struck a deal: Whenever she was feeling frayed, she was to call me, at any hour. And whenever she and my brother were truly unraveling, I'd come to provide some respite care. Never have I contributed a relatively small amount of time in a way that made such a huge difference.

You can't provide dementia care without an escape hatch or two — or ten. I've included this section because although direct-care skills are critical, you also need tools to battle the other enemies of dementia care, from pesky people and work-life conflicts to your own good intentions and the damned elusiveness of Nod.

o o o

STRESS — AND WHAT FEEDS IT

The stress of dementia care is so real you can touch it. Goodness knows, it's touching you. Study after survey shows that caregivers report more stress than non-caregivers. One report from the American Psychological Association named caregivers as one of the three most stressed groups in the land, along with the depressed and the obese. Many who provide long-term Alzheimer's care wear this Triple Crown.

Stress devastates your body and your mind. Much as I love health statistics, I'm not going to further raise your blood pressure and risk of depression by reciting all the perils here. You already know that everything from your weight and mental state to your heart health and immune system are at risk when you assume the care of another human being with dementia. Caregivers are twice as likely to smoke and 25 percent more likely to binge drink, not-so-hot coping mechanisms.

When you're stressed, the cause may seem obvious: a big medical bill, a fight with your spouse over parent care, a health scare, or all of the above. Yet the *real* stressor — the thing that sends the heart racing and the head pounding is often the way any of us *react* to a given situation. No, this doesn't mean that just thinking differently will wipe out credit card debt or make a sick person better. It means that your mental and practical responses can make or break how well you weather the storm.

As you face a given stress factor, think about what might be *really* feeding your anxiety and tension. Realizing that there's often both an immediate problem and a less obvious one can help you move toward a solution that's more constructive than alcohol, food, blood pressure meds, a day under the covers, or worse.

Five common "ultimate stressors" for caregivers include these:

Underlying stressor #1: Lack of control

You sense: "I feel stuck." "I don't have any good options." "Nobody asks what I think." "It's hopeless."

What helps: Give input and exert influence in small ways, if not large ones. When our action-oriented brains feel like we're making progress, we feel more in control.

Ask yourself:

- Can I do anything to change the situation? (Or am I stuck out of habit? Have I turned over every stone?)

- Can I assert myself more?

- Should I flat-out say no more often?

- Have I given up too easily? Who else could I talk to? Have I called the local Area Agency on Aging to find out about local resources that might be able to help?

- Have I asked my human resources office at work about resources?

- Am I moving toward a better situation, because of small changes I'm making, even if it's tough now?

Underlying stressor #2: Unrealistic expectations or standards

You sense: "Nobody can [fill in the blank] the way I do." "I'm the only one who gets it." "I should be able to manage better." "I'm always disappointed by the way they...."

What helps: Take stock of where your notions about how things "should" be or how people (including yourself) "ought" to behave came from. Much as we'd all like to be perfect, nobody — not even Mother Teresa, if you'd asked her — has reached that lofty point yet.

Ask yourself:

- Am I truly being realistic here, given the constraints of time, money, and the way this disease works?

- Why do I think something must happen a certain way?

- What would happen if it unfolded differently?

- What's the worst that could happen?

- What can I move off my to-do list by delegating, hiring help, or crossing out (spotless windows, I'm talking to you!)?

Underlying stressor #3: Uncertainty or fear

You sense: "I don't know what to expect." "How will we manage?" "What fresh hell awaits today?" "I'm terrified that things will get worse."

What helps: That old cliché "knowledge is power" also happens to be darn good advice. Reality is often frightening, to be sure. But the more you know, the more informed your perspective, and that can tamp down some of the runaway anxiety that can intensify fear.

Ask yourself:

- Have I collected enough facts?

- Have I learned about the progression of Alzheimer's — either online or in books — so I have a sense of what to expect?

- Have I made lists of questions for the doctor so I don't miss anything at appointments?

- Have I talked to other people about dementia caregiving? (Whatever your situation, you're not the first person who's gone through it.)

- Have I started making what-if plans, so that I'll be better prepared at the next juncture? Things that help include arranging the appropriate legal, financial, and advanced-care paperwork, looking into home modifications (say, for a wheelchair) or home-care aides, and exploring housing options.

- Am I looking for answers to questions that can't be answered?

- Am I worrying about what's real today and tomorrow, or getting way ahead of myself?

Underlying stressor #4: Too little self-respect

You sense: "I don't have time for myself." "With all I put up with, I deserve this pint of ice cream." "If I were stronger/more organized/more attentive, I wouldn't be so stressed out." "I hate myself."

What helps: Start by loving yourself even more than all the other people you love. That can be a tall order for the generous personality type that's often attracted to caregiving. Some caregivers suffer from "big-hearted disease," always thinking about others first. Caregivers need advocates, too — ourselves.

Ask yourself:

- Am I good to myself? Or am I doing things that make me feel better five minutes from now but will make me feel much worse in five hours? (That's the story of a bag of potato chips or a bottle of booze.)

- Am I even on my daily priority list? Or have I allowed myself to be crowded out by everyone else?

- Do I feel likeable and deserving of love? (Everyone is! But if you have trouble seeing yourself this way, it's time to find a counselor who can help you unlock this block.)

- What am I going to do for some "me" time today?

- When is the last time I had a physical exam? Do I know what my blood pressure, cholesterol levels, and other markers are saying about my own health — and am I figuring out even small ways I can optimize them? How can I arrange a short getaway — who could help me, and what do I need to do to make it happen?

Underlying stressor #5: Feeling isolated or unsupported

You sense: "Nobody understands." "They call to ask about [my mother/my father/my spouse], but never about me." "I'm too embarrassed (or depressed, or overwhelmed) to socialize."

What helps: Know that social and emotional isolation are a creeping despair that nips at all caregivers. When a situation is new or huge, we tend to hibernate. Burrowed deep in our own reality, we tend to expect others to be mind readers and see things from our vantage point, but they can't. What's more, as the disease progresses, the person with Alzheimer's often becomes unable to express gratitude. Even though you understand this intellectually, it can be hard emotionally to give and give without getting anything back.

Ask yourself:

- Have I spoken out about how I feel or what help I need?

- Am I actively seeking help, or have I been content just to grouse?

- Who's in my personal care circle? Who can I turn to for emotional support as well as for practical help? This is a new life situation and calls for a fresh support network of those who have either been there or truly get it. A few sessions with a counselor are covered by most insurance plans and can make all the difference.

- Have I called a friend or talked to one online today?

- When was the last time I got out of the house — and how can I do it again tomorrow? Look into respite programs and day programs for your loved one, so you can circulate in the world a bit.

o o o

FAMILY-RELATED STRESSORS

Criticism

Some common scenarios:

- ***Endless second-guessing:*** *One sibling is the primary caregiver. She does her best to keep the others informed—but instead of getting a sympathetic ear or reasoned input, they question her every decision: "Why this medication and not that one?" "I've heard a better thing to do is…." "That lawyer is a crook; you should have used a different one."*

- ***Sharing problems but no solutions:*** *Some people like to point out what's wrong without offering a better way. Nutrition, socialization, hygiene, finances — any topic of care is fair game. Often, of course, the hands-on caregiver is well aware of a problem or a situation that's less than ideal (mom hates getting a bath, the local day program is too expensive). She wants help, not a restatement of the obvious.*

- ***Laying blame:*** *Some people need a demon. Rather than blaming the disease for taking away a loved one, they project their distress on the primary caregiver. Situations that are nobody's 'fault" get unfairly pinned on the caregiver: "You let him wander away — where were you?" "She's in the hospital again?" "How did she get these bedsores?"*

What you should know about criticism:

Fault-finders often operate on auto-pilot. It's their reflexive way of seeing the world. And when they're feeling guilty or insecure, it's as if they go on a finger-pointing mission. Unconsciously, they're asking themselves, *How can I make you feel bad so I feel better?* Judgmental people tend to pick on the handiest scapegoat they can find. The perfect target: a relative or friend whom they perceive as being closer to the person with Alzheimer's, or doing more, or knowing more.

Devaluing someone else through shame or blame makes a critic feel superior (even if it isn't true), relieving their insecurity, guilt, or low self esteem — at least temporarily.

Criticism isn't always a psychological power play, of course. The critic may intend to be helpful, not hurtful, in a clumsy way; maybe she's a Type A personality who sees something that needs fixing and can't help herself, for example. Sometimes criticisms are made off-the-cuff, the thoughtless comments or uninformed questions of someone who sees the dementia only in small doses and doesn't have a real sense of what you're going through. Before you get your hackles up, consider whether the critic "gets" what's going on.

And, of course, if the criticisms are coming from someone with dementia, you have to factor this in to your response. Hearing such digs is every bit as deflating as when they come from someone else, but the origin is different. A person with Alzheimer's who criticizes and complains is usually doing so out of disease-triggered fear or insecurity. They're not comparing themselves to you or looking to build themselves up by tearing you down.

What can help you:

- **Use "I" statements that play back how the hurtful words make you feel:** "I feel hurt when you talk to me like that." "I really feel upset when you criticize every decision I make." "I feel uncomfortable around you because I never know when your criticisms are coming or why you make them." When you say you're hurt by a critic's words, it's paralyzing to him. Talking about feelings zaps the emotional distance such people like to keep between themselves and others, which makes it easier to keep on criticizing.

- **Sidestep getting roped into further judgments on your character.** Bullies often respond with comments like, "Oh, you're too sensitive!" "I'm only trying to help if you'd let me!" It's a way of masking their pushiness by turning it back on you. Say, "I can't help my reaction." "I'd like your help, but your tone is hurtful and unproductive."

- **Don't argue the issue.** You only give a fault-finder an excuse to justify the criticism and belittle you further. You're much more empowered if you can turn the discussion away from the critic's perceptions of you to your own feelings.

- **Turn their words back on them.** Without arguing, try to move the conversation in a more constructive direction: "What can *you* do to change that?" "That's an interesting opinion, tell me what you'd do differently and how." (These tips don't always work with a really toxic critic, so if you're not hearing true help, abandon this strategy.)

- **Don't let yourself believe what you hear.** A criticism carries two parts — the perceived fault ("You let Dad wander off!") and the hidden meaning implied ("therefore you're a jerk!"). What a chronic fault-finder is really saying is that it's not just your behavior that's the problem — it's the meaning of it. "If you choose not to buy into the 'that makes me bad,' part, you're inoculated against the dart; it's not going to hurt you," says psychotherapist Steve Sultanoff, an adjunct professor at Pepperdine University.

- **Don't apologize automatically if you're not in the wrong.** ("Oh, sorry, sorry!") That doesn't smooth things over; it only feeds bullying behavior. Better: Stand up for yourself.

- **If the criticisms seem to stem from well-intentioned ignorance,** invite the critic to spend more time with the person who has dementia, such as subbing for you while you run errands or taking over weekend care. There's nothing like hands-on experience to make someone see a situation differently.

- **Applaud yourself and all you do.** Talking yourself down ("I'm fat," "I'm bad at talking to doctors") is just piling on. Pep talk that's positive might feel corny ("Nice reply!" "Good hair day!") but has been shown to actually make you feel better. Hey, if you're constantly being taken down by others, you owe it to yourself to look out for Number One.

- **Keep your distance.** Ultimately, your health comes first. You're well within your rights to avoid someone who only wants to level you, especially if they do nothing in the way of balancing their snipes with practical, emotional, or financial support.

- **Listen for a nugget of truth.** Criticism isn't always unfounded or unwarranted. Try to listen neutrally, with an open mind, to see if there's anything eye opening or useful you can pluck from what at first sounds like an attack. After all, people have different values, life experiences, contacts, and other influences on how they react to different situations. Ask yourself what they must be seeing through the lens of their experience to make them say what they did. If you think a remark is accurate, or contains useful help, say so, say thanks, and move on.

o o o

Denial

Some common scenarios:

- ***Problem, what problem?*** *After my mom fell and broke her pelvis, and the degree of my dad's worsening dementia became obvious, my siblings and I began to discuss their living situation after the immediate crisis ended. To some of us, it seemed obvious that their days of living independently without any kind of help were numbered. What should we do? But some siblings weren't convinced. They said things like, "This is just a short-term problem...Let's not get ahead of ourselves... Dad's just getting older...."*

- ***Making excuses:*** *Some people would rather blame anything other than Alzheimer's for what's going on: age, recovery from surgery, orneriness, disorientation from a move, etc. There may be a few grains of truth in there. Unfortunately such an attitude gets in the way of getting everyone on board to do things like protect finances, curb dangerous driving, start medications or other therapies, and so on.*

- ***Too close for discomfort.*** *The person who's nearest to the one with cognitive trouble — a spouse, the adult child who lives next-door — sometimes has more denial than more distant family. Those who are farther away often have the advantage of noticing changes more immediately. To someone who's there every day, incremental changes can be less visible.*

- ***Self-denial.*** *It's not uncommon for caregivers to have an unrealistic sense of the situation they're in. They think they can do it alone, for example, or put up with situations long after they're unsafe. Those with a martyr bent to their personality, with a large capacity for suffering beyond what many healthy people would consider tolerable, can cling to a warped perception of reality for a long time.*

- ***Denial by owner:*** *The person in denial is sometimes the person with dementia. Early in the disease, when awareness is still intact,* *the person may refuse to admit anything's amiss — or just refuse to talk about it.*

What you should know about denial:

Denial — refusing to face facts — is usually rooted in fear. Someone in denial may be afraid of what's ahead, known or unknown. So like the proverbial ostrich with its head in the sand, it becomes easier not to see a problem than to face it.

For some, the stakes are too high to face reality. They have too much vested in their own illusion of the way things are now. ("I'm busy in my career; I'm sure Dad and Mom are fine on their own." "I still feel like a kid myself; my father can't be losing it yet!") That version of reality might not be logical, but they cling to it.

Another contributing factor: Alzheimer's can be so startling and strange that we're willing to consider any other explanation for what's going on, no matter how implausible. Some people will even turn a problem into a fault of yours ("Why are you looking for trouble?") rather than see a situation that needs addressing.

It may feel good to be in denial, but the dangers are multifold:

- Denial can get in the way of getting good care or making a situation safer. Many families make excuses ("it's not that bad...") until the person is lost on the highway, having driven across three state lines.

- Denial can make everyday life harder. If you don't see a situation realistically, you're less likely to get sufficient help. You might hold onto expectations for how your loved one should behave and wind up chronically disappointed or exhausted.

- Denial can strain relationships. When one person isn't even seeing the problem, it's hard to strategize together about a solution.

- Denial can interfere with quality of life. This is often seen at the end of life, when families are resistant to discuss hospice or palliative care because they're in denial about the specter of death. Instead of a peaceful last chapter, there may be intrusive hospitalizations and family disagreement.

It's important to realize that although people who are sick are often in denial about their condition, Alzheimer's presents a different type of denial. Someone with Alzheimer's eventually lacks the capacity to have an awareness of what's going on in his own brain. This kind of denial is especially challenging for a caregiver, because it requires a different set of skills to deal with it.

What can help you:

- **Give a denier a little space.** Denial can be a shock absorber for the soul, a coping mechanism that allows people to maintain sanity and get used to a change. Some people need more time than others to face the realities of a difficult situation.

- **Decide how much someone else's denial is a problem for you.** Some denial gets in the way of help. Other times it's just vexing because it means others don't agree with you — but doesn't really affect your day-to-day life.

- **Separate denial from lack of knowledge.** Denial is refusing to acknowledge facts — but you have to have the facts in the first place. Be sure that the person having a hard time accepting a situation at least understands the options, symptoms, treatments, or other relevant information. Present the full story, with all the relevant facts. Share informative books or articles. Encourage conversations with doctors, other experts, or friends who have been in similar situations.

- **Calmly repeat the facts as necessary.** Without being judgmental, review reality as you understand it: "Mom,

Dad is repeating himself every five minutes. You told me yourself he made three big mistakes with the bills over the last three months. The neighbor had to lead him home from the grocery last week. These are big changes for him, and I think the doctor should hear about them and see what he thinks." Sometimes making a written list of relevant facts helps.

- **Don't take anyone's denial personally.** It may cause the other person to criticize your judgment or accuse you of overreacting, but if you're confident of the truth, take comfort in that and keep your ego out of the dispute.

- **Encourage talk about the very thing that's being avoided.** Probe gently: "Why do you think Mom will be able to live alone in this two-story house when the doctor said she won't be able to walk again?" "What would be the worst that would happen if we talked to someone from hospice, just to learn more about it?"

- **Probe with hypotheticals:** It's easier for some people to imagine "pretend" situations rather than the ones they currently see. "What if Mom's mistakes with driving the car continue; what will happen? I'd hate it if she got hurt or hurt someone." "I know you think Dad doesn't have a urinary tract infection, but what if it is? What would that mean? Maybe we should find out." These scenarios can nudge the person along in his or her thinking.

- **Record visual proof. Some people in denial are persuaded by hard evidence.** Make a video of your dad limping: "See how hard it is for him to walk?" It can be especially persuasive if you can compare it to an earlier recording. Or tape a conversation with your mom showing her confusion that you can play later for siblings: "See? I'm not making this up!"

- **Don't confuse denial with giving up hope.** Having hope means you're moving forward based on a clear grasp of reality: the dire as well as the unknowable, maybe seasoned with faith. Hope is a commodity that most people feel is a help, not a hindrance, and one that needn't be abandoned in any situation. Denial, in

267

contrast, means avoiding reality because it's too painful to behold — which usually also means denying help (such as stronger pain meds, more adult day care, the comfort of assisted living, or palliative care).

o o o

Disagreement

Some common scenarios:

- *How to pay for care and other financial matters:* Money matters are a top source of discord. One sibling wants to sell the family home; the other feels everything possible should be done to keep Mom in familiar surroundings. A well-to-do sibling expects the others to do their share. Spouses disagree over the terms of a will.

- **Medical conundrums:** To operate or not to operate? This medication or that one? Participate in a clinical trial or no? When the patient in question can't reliably make his own decisions, families may not agree on what he'd prefer or what's in his best interest. Often there isn't one "right" answer.

- **Mom always liked you best!** Disagreements can have deep roots. When our birth families are involved, we often revert back to childhood roles, and with them, the slights and perceptions that were formed during those years. Charges of favoritism can cause arguments. So can birth order's built-in expectations, such as the eldest expecting the younger sibs to go along with him, or that the youngest has no idea what she's talking about.

- **It's not your business!** A wife dealing with her husband's memory problems might not like what her daughter has to say about the matter. A live-in caregiver feels she has a different perspective from her sister who lives 100 miles away. A stepson's opinion is valued less than a son's, even though the two were practically raised together.

What you should know about disagreement:

All families argue. Whether your relations over the years have been generally harmonious or always cantankerous, you can count on the fact that dealing with Alzheimer's is going to create friction. If you've always had problems, they're apt to intensify. If you've never had discord before, get ready.

That's partly because you're in a situation where emotions run high. Many decisions, large and small, must be made about care, living situation, independence, medical condition, and that ever-discordant topic (whether Alzheimer's is present or not), money. Everyone involved has his or her own values, life experiences, and unique relationship with the person affected. You may be as close as can be with Dad, but your stepmother, your husband, and your daughter each have their own very personal relationship. The same facts can look surprisingly different from each vantage point.

The trick is to manage discord before it eats away at you or your relationships and gets in the way of your loved one's care.

Arguments are often fed by some of the other stressors discussed in this chapter: resentment, depression, and favoritism, for example.

What can help you:

- **Agree to disagree.** First, realize that there are some issues where everyone won't be on board, and that's okay. Separate the small stuff from the biggies.

- **Keep everyone in the loop as best you can.** Sometimes people quibble because they're not up to date on the facts or they're objecting to being left out. For some families, family meetings (ideally, including the person with Alzheimer's) serve this purpose. Other ways to do this include conference calls (many services provide toll-free numbers), email updates, private Facebook pages, or online care-circle services. Keeping written records of expenditures, health, and resources used (even if they go ignored by family) puts things in black and white, which can help insulate you in the unfortunate event of later attacks.

- **Keep the focus squarely on the person in need.** Relationships are complex. Emotions run high. Ask yourself if you're locked in a showdown over the problem or over personalities. Sometimes what can seem like a disagreement over how to proceed is really a reactionary push-me-pull-you tug-of-war in which one party just can't stand for the other one to be right. Remind siblings (or adult children): "This is about Mom; it's not about me or you."

- **Ask, "What do you think?"** Try stepping back from pushing your point of view and ask for advice. Even if you think the advice is wrong, just listen. This approach can disarm someone who wants to tangle and break the fight dynamic, allowing you to move to a more collaborative plane.

- **Divide and conquer.** You don't have to all agree or contribute in equal measure. In many families, members have different domains of expertise. Among my own siblings, for example, a sister in the insurance business managed the paperwork. A builder brother handled household repairs and modifications. I held the medical power of attorney and took care of interactions with doctors. My older sister was good at moral support and hands-on care. We compared notes on the big stuff but mostly let each person make smaller decisions within his or her area of knowledge. This approach has the added advantage of lightening the workload, so it doesn't all fall on one person. (My mom, a single child, used to say that the silver lining in caring for her mother's long decline with Alzheimer's was that at least she didn't have to argue with anybody else about her decisions.)

- **Get the help of a mediator.** Professional elder mediators are a terrific resource, especially when big decisions (about where to live, how to spend money, taking away the car keys, or major medical decisions) are tearing a family apart. Mediators cut stress and help families move forward by creating a safe and neutral space for all parties to be heard and for the interests of the person with dementia to be kept in view. They're also skilled at hammering out an action plan for a solution — so you don't just end the bickering but actually move forward. Mediators can be especially helpful where one party is crying foul, or when suspicions about finances and motives have been raised.

Ask your local Area Agency on Aging or a geriatric care

manager or lawyer to recommend mediators who specialize in eldercare or gerontology, or check the local services directory at Caring.com. You'll spend a little money (rates average around $150/hour) but can actually save in the end, because a caregiver's time and sanity are too valuable to squander in spinning your wheels debating with family.

o o o

Favoritism

Some common scenarios:

- *The swoop-in, swoop-out superhero.* Sibling A lives near her parents and is there day-in, day-out helping with everything from doctor appointments to medication reminders. She feels taken for granted. Sibling B lives across the country — swoops in twice a year to visit and dazzles the parents with her attention and care. Never mind that she then disappears after stirring up half-baked plans and hopes, seldom to be heard from until the next hero's welcome.

- *The halo effect.* *Sometimes one sibling Can Do No Wrong and the other...well, it doesn't matter how many "rights" he or she says and does. Often a parent will defer to the eldest, or to a son over a daughter, or to the child who lives closest.*

- *Old wounds.* *A perceived rivalry can be rooted in decades-old competitive feelings...he always let you get away with things...she gets more because she's the baby...Dad never took me seriously....*

- *Sibling Olympics.* *Some hyper-competitive siblings strive to out-care one another. They duke it out for recognition as Most Dutiful Daughter, undermining one another's efforts along the way. Mom or Dad agrees with whomever they last talked to. Although it's much more common to have too few devoted caregivers, rather than too many, any situation where everyone's not on the same page can be dangerous.*

What you should know about favoritism:

Can you say infuriating? Of course you can if you feel that you're a bypassed sibling. You can feel it, taste it, and touch it.

The favoritism may be real or only seem that way. Perception is a big part of the problem. But parents do show preferences. Research has recently debunked the idealized notion that mothers don't have favorites. Purdue's J. Jill Suitor and Cornell's Karl Pillemer, both sociologists, did a series of studies with hundreds of women ages 65 to 75. Most admitted feeling emotionally closest to daughters (four times more often than sons) and youngest children. In a crisis, though, they'd turn to a first-born for advice. Perceived favoritism ripples all through life, say Suitor and Pillemer. Those who sensed it growing up tend to grapple more with depression as adults.

And here's the really interesting part: When the women were re-interviewed at 72 and 82, the one they'd felt closest to wound up playing caregiver three-quarters of the time. But when a different child fell into that role, the mothers were more often depressed. Research published by Pillemer in 2013 shows that the preferred child tends to share values with the mother, live nearby, and yes, be a daughter.

To some degree, it's a like-it-or-lump-it situation, because you can't change your parents' feelings or how you feel about them. The difficulty is that these perceptions can get in the way of giving someone with Alzheimer's the best possible care (and protecting your own health and sense of self-worth).

The going can get roughest when it seems like there's disparity over:

- Finances. Who "gets" more or is being dealt a fair hand gets tangled in the roots of childhood rivalry, which is a craving for equal love and attention from parents. And, very sad to say, some people get greedy as a relative grows more infirm.

- Legal influence. Fears over who's exacting the most control over health care decisions or legal-financial decisions get dicey, because powers of attorney are often held by one person, rather than shared.

- An uneven burden of care. It's bad enough to do the lion's share of work; it's harder when you feel like someone who does less is rewarded more.

The dynamics can get trickier when adult siblings don't even know one another very well. It's not uncommon for kids to grow up, move away, and have few day-to-day dealings with one another. They never develop adult relationships. They're stuck in old childhood ways of interacting (often featuring lots of immature competition and bickering).

Parents, too, may not have strong or realistic adult-to-adult relationships with grown children. They may fall into old patterns that serve neither party well. Then, when a crisis hits that requires everyone to pull together and communicate, everyone's ill-equipped to do so.

What can help you:

- **Be sure you're assessing a situation realistically.** Are your hackles up because of what's being done (or not done) or because you're reacting to some personality trait or pattern in a sibling? You may well be in the right, but it's important to separate past grudges from what's best in the present situation.

- **Talk about your roles in concrete ways.** "Rivalries re-emerge because we no longer know who is who in our family, or at least, who does what," notes Francine Russo in *They're Your Parents, Too,* her guide to sibling relationships in eldercare. It can help to step back from your assumptions. Talk together about how weird this dynamic is. Say, okay, who's going to gather which information? How are we going to make decisions? What do we do when we can't agree?

- **Focus on the big picture.** It's common, and easy, to resent someone who comes in from afar to stir things up and give glamorous input when you're the one who does the dirty work day-in, day-out. Try not to take it personally that their relatively small efforts are applauded while yours go unrecognized. (Yes, it's especially rankling when the hero-for-a-day doesn't acknowledge all you do.)

- **Try bringing in outside help.** If everyone agrees, try meeting with a geriatric care manager or an eldercare mediator (a family mediator with expertise in aging issues). These impartial experts are skilled at cutting through the layers of familial sediment and impediment. Try using the argument that you're all in this for the long haul (the rest of your lives), and a neutral third-party can both do what's best for your loved one and preserve your future relationships.

o o o

Lack of Family Help

Some common scenarios:

- *All talk, no action.* *"Let me know if I can help!" says the relative. But when you ask, the would-be helper is inevitably busy that day. Or worse, she cancels at the last minute. Her life always takes priority over yours.*

- *Out of sight, out of mind.* *Family members who aren't on the scene seem to simply vanish. They might call and ask how the person with Alzheimer's is doing, in a perfunctory way, but they never bother to ask how you're holding up. Or they just assume you have things covered and vamoose.*

- *Not my thing.* *Some people have really creative reasons for not being able to help: "It makes me sad to see him this way." "I'm just not very good around old people." "It would be too depressing/ too stressful/ too upsetting for me." "I'm not in the best of health myself you know; I have migraines." "I'd rather remember him the way he used to be." (Yes, these are all real excuses family caregivers have reported hearing!)*

What you should know about lack of help:

The bottom line: People either want to help you or they don't.

Often people want to lend a hand but hang back for legitimate reasons. They may not be sure how to offer their assistance or what kind would make a difference. When they offer, a caregiver may fall into that social-niceness dance of shrugging it off, and then the helper doesn't persist. Some people do feel awkward around older adults or those with Alzheimer's — even close family members — and can benefit from a little hand-holding and education. It can also help to give them chores that are less hands-on but just as beneficial to you. Ironically, some caregivers make their tasks look so easy (and complain so little) that family members don't even suspect they're needed.

But if there's one truism about help when caring for someone with Alzheimer's, it's that more is always better.

Sadly, some people really don't want to help. It may have to do with their own internal conflicts, problems, or feelings about the person with Alzheimer's, or it could have to do with their relationship to you. You may never know.

What can help you:

- **Make lists!** Write down everything you must do to run your life and manage care. When someone asks how she can help, whip out the list and ask back, "Great, what would you like to do?"

- **Get a firm commitment.** Well-intentioned helpers are themselves helped when you give specific tasks at specific times. They'll be more likely to follow through.

- **Set up repeat gigs.** Your nephew driving your mom to a hair appointment is great. Having him do it every month? Invaluable.

- **Remember that "help" has many definitions.** Because I'm self-employed, it was easy for me to be the respite caregiver for my dad during the time he lived with my brother a couple of hours away. In between, I made a point of calling my sister-in-law often just to be a sounding board and source of stress release. She also knew she could call me at any hour (and did!). It was a small thing on my part, but sometimes the difference between going bonkers and holding on another day is a small thing.

- **Don't waste precious time and emotional energy beating your head against a wall.** If family members rebuff you repeatedly, give up. Yes, I said give up. Sometimes you have to "accept what you cannot change" and let go of the resentment, anger, and frustration that builds up when those who ought to step up instead choose to step back. Your emotional energy is valuable.

Spend it on making life better for your loved one — and yourself — in the ways that are in your control.

- **Look outside the family circle.** When family won't help, redouble your efforts to tap into community resources that can, starting with the clearinghouse Area Agency on Aging.

- **Shore up personal support for yourself.** A support group can offer hive-mind problem solving and idea sharing, along with opportunities to vent a little, which caregivers forced into lone-soldier syndrome especially need.

- **Be sure you're not part of the problem.** Some caregivers wind up as Lone Rangers because that's exactly how they set things up. They fail to reach out to others when it's needed. Or they rebuff help that's offered. They don't want to "bother" anyone. Let go of old ideas that asking for help is a sign of weakness. If ever you needed other people in your life, it's now.

Caregivers may also fall into the rut of believing that nobody can do it as well as they can, notes AARP family expert Amy Goyer. Gail Sheehy, author of *Passages in Caregiving,* calls this "playing God" — she says she felt personally responsible for warding off all disasters and dangers. While it's true in many cases that the hands-on caregiver does the best job of providing care, a nobody-can-do-it-like-me attitude ultimately doesn't add up to the common good. You need help. Most people like to help. Your loved one with Alzheimer's will manage just fine under someone else's temporary watch. Remember, too, that people can help you out in ways that don't replicate your hands-on caregiving efforts. They can help you manage your life or your stress load, handle paperwork, drive to appointments, and so on.

o o o

Relationship Strain

Some common scenarios:

- *Honor thy parent or thy partner first?* *Caring for a parent with dementia can take a lot of time — leaving one's spouse to feel resentful, even abandoned.*

- *I am sandwich filling.* *The average caregiver is a woman in her late 40s to early 50s — prime time to still have children in school as along with aging parents with health issues. She feels constantly torn between the two generations. (Men experience this, too.) Children may complain of feeling neglected or begin to act out in ways that test limits.*

- *Peter, Pammy, and Polly Pan.* *In a crisis, it's a typical dynamic for adult children to revert to their childhood roles and perceptions of one another. A successful lawyer born last remains the "baby" and sibs can't even take her legal advice seriously. Or the oldest is expected to make the hard decisions. Or the wild "black sheep" is left out of everything.*

- *Family rifts.* *Caregiving situations can bring out ugly undercurrents with immediate or extended family. There may be disagreements about money, suspicions over motives, and disappointments over actions (or lack of actions).*

- *Fair-weather friends.* *You get busy, they can't relate — and before you know it, there's a gulf between you and your friends.*

What you should know about relationship strain:

Conflicts with the other people in your life are incredibly common. Alzheimer's doesn't just affect the person with the disease — everyone in his or her circle is touched, as are, in turn, the relatives and friends in *your* circle.

Fully 80 percent of caregivers report that caregiving strained their marriage or other key relationships, found a 2009 Caring.com survey. Half of caregivers say that their duties take time away from friends and other family members, according to the National Alliance for Caregiving (NAC). And about a third of caregivers say that their emotions interfere "a lot" with their social lives, found a 2011 UCLA Center for Health Policy report.

And it all happens almost without you realizing it. "The risk of caregiving is that you gravitate toward newness — you have to pay attention to every new situation or crisis," says Carol D. O'Dell, a Florida-based speaker on caregiving who took care of her mom for 10 years and author of *Mothering Mother.* "And you ignore all the quieter people and situations in your life."

Net result: isolation, tension, resentment, a perceived lack of support, lost sources of support — and a lot more stress in an already overstressed life. Caregivers who sacrifice time with family and friends are more than twice as likely to feel stress as those who preserve time with others, says the NAC data.

What can help you:

- **Consciously decide that others matter.** This is a problem where sheer awareness helps. It's easy to get so focused on your loved one with Alzheimer's that you take others for granted. In a crisis, that's inevitable. But you can't let crisis become chronic, because everyone needs you to some extent — and you need them. Keep a mental tally of the people who matter, and make a point of checking in. It never pays to take someone for granted for too long — including (or maybe especially) a beloved spouse.

- **Talk about your distraction.** Let them know that you know your presence has been scarce or conflicted. Try saying things like, "I can tell you're not happy now, and neither am I. I know things can't be exactly the same as they once were between us, right now, but let's work together to try harder."

- **Set up rituals that bring you together.** When your time and attention are at a premium, it can help to "institutionalize" together time — make it part of your daily routine. Maybe you get up early to have breakfast with your teen before school or take an after-dinner walk with your spouse while your mom dozes.

- **Don't make false assumptions.** When you're deep in Alzheimer's care, others' issues and interests can seem more trivial. To you, perhaps they are — but they're not to the person having them. Make a concerted effort to ask about the challenges and concerns facing your loved ones. Stay in the game — maybe not to your usual extent but enough to show you care. Maybe you can't have a weekly lunch date, but you can text or send birthday cards, for example.

- **Avoid forming unrealistic expectations**. It would be nice if everyone understood how difficult and consuming Alzheimer's care can be. But they don't. Even a long-loved spouse who lives under the same roof as you may not be completely on the same page. A teenager may adore Grandpa, but developmentally, it's normal for her to see herself as the center of her own universe, not her grandfather. You have to accept that this is okay and let it go. If you're constantly expecting people to pitch in or lend an ear in ways they're not, you'll constantly be disappointed and nursing a hurt.

- **Outgrow old expectations.** Is someone locked into thinking a younger sibling is too immature to make decisions (even though she's 35)? Or that a son should manage money while a daughter manages doctor appointments? Gender stereotypes and childhood roles can get in the way of having good relationships now. Gently remind someone stuck in this kind of thinking that you're all grown-ups now.

- **Find solace in those who "know."** Support groups or online chat groups can be a kind of pressure valve for your primary relationships. When you can blow off steam to those who *do* know what you're going through, you're apt to be more emotionally available to, and more tolerant of, these other loved ones.

- **Sometimes, you just have to let them go.** It's not unusual for some friends or family to fall away due to the stress of caregiving. You might reunite later, or you might not. If a relationship can't stand up to being on the back burner temporarily, or if arguments are too corrosive, step back. Let the relationship die a natural death. Just be cautious not to do this with *all* your relationships simply because it feels easier. You need a support network now more than ever. Even when you're stressed, connection works both ways.

o o o

EMOTIONAL STRESSORS

When You Feel Guilty

Some common stressors:

- *Guilt for what I'm not doing.* I should be entertaining Grandma more...I should cook healthier meals...I ought to get us both exercising...

- *Guilt for what I'm doing.* I feel bad that I have to take him to the day center, but I need a break...I shouldn't rush through her shower like that...I ought to be able to handle this without whining — after all I'm her daughter!

- *Guilt for not doing enough.* After years of struggles, one caregiver agonized over whether it was time to place her diabetic and demented mom, who was obese and becoming incontinent, into a care facility. When her mom needed an amputation, the discharge planner and doctors agreed there was little question that this would be best. A good option was found that worked out well all around. But the caregiver nevertheless felt she had let her mother down. "I feel like there's more I could have done...."

- *Guilt for being away.* Long-distance caregivers feel their cash and phone support isn't enough. Those who use respite care are pricked with feelings of insufficiency because they can't do it 24/7.

- *Guilt for being happy or well.* "I'm in a good mood today — oh wait, I shouldn't be, because my husband is sick." "Why am I the healthy one and he's in such terrible shape?"

What you should know about guilt:

As the examples illustrate, there's no end to opportunities for guilt in the realm of caregiving. You can't ignore this pesky emotion. You can't will it away. Guilt simply *is*.

Occasionally guilt can be a productive emotion. Call it "good guilt" — the nagging voice in our heads that causes us to examine our behavior and decide whether a change is in order. If you feel guilty because you were impatient with your loved one, for example, it's like a little poke reminding you to try harder or take a deep breath next time. Guilty you didn't go to the gym? Yes, that would have been good for you, and what would make that possible?

Unfortunately most of what eats us alive is "bad guilt." Bad guilt has no constructive underbelly. Bad guilt makes you feel bad about a situation that you can't help (your parent has to move to rehab, for instance) or that is actually a positive for you (you've hired home care because you can't do it all yourself).

Then we beat ourselves up for reasons that are unrealistic and counterproductive. All that stewing and self-flagellation wastes precious mental energy.

(If you're a mother, you're probably a champion at guilt. Women who are actively being caregiving to both a parent and children at the same time are the squishy-squashy filling of triple-decker guilt sandwiches.)

What can help you:

- **Beware the "red flag words":** *Ought to, should, could have, always, never.* Ban them from your vocabulary; they're warnings that you're setting the bar too high. When you hear yourself saying, "I should..." flick your forefinger against your wrist as a reminder. "Always" and "never" are toxic because they set us up for future guilt: "I'll never put you in a home." "I'll always be here." Don't promise things you can't be 100 percent certain of — most things in life!

- **Don't discount yourself.** Ironically, selfless people (the dominant caregiver personality) tend to feel proportionately more guilt. Because they work so hard aspiring to an ideal of doing things for others, they tend to ignore the inconvenient reality that they have to look after themselves all the more. They may even forget that they, too, deserve extras and shortcuts and breaks. When they finally get around to a slow bath or a lunch with friends, it feels as alien as it does great. Trust your needs, your perceptions, your value in this situation.

- **Aim to be a B+ caregiver.** Straight As are for grad students and crazoids, not mere mortals with houses to keep, relationships to tend, jobs to do, and sanity to uphold. No caregiver anticipates every fall or prevents every bedsore. Tempers boil. Germs sneak in. Bills slip through unpaid. In other words, life happens. No matter how much you love the person or feel you "owe" him or her, you'll all be happier if you lower your standards to the level of real life. By aiming for the B, you'll achieve good marks consistently, and occasionally surprise yourself with an A, rather than constantly feeling like you're missing the mark.

- **Remind yourself of your true goals here.** Ideally, you should be striving to give your loved one a secure life free of worry or pain, while maintaining your own quality of life and health. Don't beat yourself up over the small stuff.

- **Steer clear of comparisons.** We feel guilt when we feel that we're falling short of some imagined ideal. Where do those ideas come from? Often, from our own heads. We compare ourselves to someone else, without stopping to calculate what their stress levels or support situation is like, without allowing that every case is different. It doesn't matter if Nancy Reagan seemed like a saint over her husband's disease but all you want to do is cry and complain. Were you inside their house, seeing what went on? All that matters is you and yours, and how to make your hard situation as easy as you can.

- **See it as a sign of strength, not weakness, to enlist help.** Strong, smart people know that Alzheimer's care is not a task for the isolated and solitary. The more you can delegate and share, the better life feels. Only those with too much hubris and willful ignorance of reality think they can do it by themselves. And when strong, smart people get help, they don't look back and feel guilty about it.

- **Get the doctor's (or a therapist's) ten cents.** There's nothing like hearing from a neutral third party, "No, you have nothing to feel guilty about in that situation." Often we don't believe the obvious unless we hear if from a trusted, neutral source.

Photocopy and post these promises to yourself:

1. I'll apologize when I lose my temper, but I realize that caregiving is so chock-full of temperature-riling situations that eternal calm is impossible.

2. I'll be there for my loved one, but I'll continue to run my own life at the same time.

3. I'll let myself grieve and cry and feel sad instead of trying to keep a chipper smile on my face all the time.

4. I'll accept or ignore criticism for what it's worth (or not worth) rather than letting it eat at me.

5. I'll quit blaming myself when bad things happen. Bad things happen.

6. I resolve to take care of *me*, not just my loved one. Because eventually I may be the one who needs care, and better it be later than sooner.

o o o

When You Feel Resentful

Some common scenarios:

- *Why me? Resenting others.* You avoid Facebook because you're tired of reading about your friends' latest vacations and new cars. Relatives with big jobs go off to important offices every day. Everyone else seems to be living life to the fullest, while your days feel small and full of obligations.

- *Not the way it was supposed to be: resenting fate.* "We were supposed to retire to the lake house." "I took care of the house and kids all those years, and now this was supposed to be my time." "I'm too young for this." "Other girls get to have their dads walk them down the aisle at their weddings; mine is in a nursing home with early onset Alzheimer's." "My wife spends all her time caring for her parents; what about me and our life?"

- *I love you and I hate you. Resenting the person with Alzheimer's.* "I'm just so tired of this." "Why didn't you take better care of yourself?" "Why didn't you tell me you were having trouble earlier?" "Why are you so difficult and ungrateful?" "Why do you blame me when I'm the one trying to help you????"

What you should know about resentment:

Resentment is the "dirty little secret" emotion of caregiving. It's such a complex and taboo topic that few people readily cop to it. Yet it's an all-too-common feeling and tends to ramp up the more hands-on the care you provide and the longer that caregiving goes on.

Why shouldn't we resent a role none of us asked for and for which few of us have any real preparation? You may have volunteered to be a caregiver, but nobody asks for Alzheimer's. It's not only perfectly plausible, but natural, to love someone, care well for him or her, even continue to treasure moments together — and still resent the hijacked course your lives have taken because of this particularly insidious disease. Resentment can co-exist alongside other emotions.

The dark side of resentment is that it can raise your blood pressure, shorten your temper, sap your energy, and lead you to drink, smoke, or relieve stress in other unhealthy ways. Not so good.

On the brighter side, having an awareness of your feelings — even the darkest ones — is the first step toward better health and can help improve your overall situation.

What can help you:

- **Start by acknowledging your resentment.** Give yourself permission to *have* this difficult emotion. It's okay. Resenting the fix you're in doesn't make you a bad person — it makes you a candid one.

- **Vent safely about it.** What's challenging about resentment is finding outlets that won't judge you or recoil in horror when you admit to it. A trusted friend to whom you can say anything is invaluable. But failing that, turn to support groups, a therapist, or online caregiver networks. Scribble your feelings in a journal — and then, if you want, rip them up or burn them afterward.

- **Try to avoid making comparisons.** This is really hard, but resentment tends to intensify when you compare one life to another — yours to your siblings, your past to your present, your long-dreamed future to your likely realistic one.

- **Be galvanized, rather than paralyzed, by resentment.** Consider these prickly feelings as a personal message system. Use them as a warning that you should find more resources for help, enlist others in ways large and small, defend your health, and take other steps that will improve your day-to-day existence.

- **Revisit the big picture every now and then.** A given hour, day, or week might be especially awful. Step back and look at the full arc of your life — past and future. It won't change what you're going through but can grant you a perspective that makes it more bearable.

o o o

When You Lose Your Temper or Patience

Some common scenarios:

- *Taking it out on your loved one:* It used to startle me to hear my mother snap at my dad. When the phone rang, he might pick up one of the three TV remotes and say "Hello!" into it. (He had dementia, but those long black devices did all look similar!) "Not that one, the other one!" Mom would hiss at him — as if it hadn't happened a hundred times before.

- *Taking it out on a third party:* Out of the blue, you yell at your child, just because she left her shoes on the floor. Or you call the girl at the drive-thru window a name because she forgot to put napkins in your bag. Told on the phone that you can't get your preferred appointment time, you erupt into full Mount MisplacedAngerSuvius.

What you should know about anger and impatience:

Everybody "loses it" sometimes. It may not be a particularly attractive human quality, but it's a natural act. And in the Alzheimer's caregiving setting, it might even be an inevitable one.

Anger often seems like it's being tripped by what's happening at the moment: a mistake, a balky loved one, a criticism, a mishap. But typically the incident is just the proverbial straw that breaks your back. There are usually underlying factors that are simmering beneath the surface. These can include chronic stress, lack of sleep, frustration over lack of control, grief, or disappointments that have little direct connection to the meltdown.

"Stress rolls downhill" is how Oprah's favorite life coach, Martha Beck, refers to this displaced aggression. We tend to dump our anger on someone else, usually someone we know won't fight back.

Blowing up lets you release a little steam, momentarily. It's not the best way to let off steam, but it works — which is why we keep doing it.

Beware, though: Chronic anger and hostility are linked to high blood pressure, heart attack and heart disease, digestive tract disorders, and headaches. Anger that builds and *doesn't* get expressed can lead to depression or anxiety. Anger that explodes outwardly can jeopardize relationships and even cause harm. That's why finding good ways to manage caregiver anger helps both you and the person in your care.

What can help you:

When you slip:

- For the occasional blooper, forgive yourself and forget. Seriously.

- Apologize to the injured party with a little self-blame: "I'm so sorry. I don't know where that came from — well, I do; I've just been under a lot of stress. It's my fault, not yours." Or, "Sorry! That was the stress talking! It's about me, not you!"

- Vow to try harder next time. Patience really is a virtue, which is what makes it a worthy goal — even if not always an attainable one.

- If you find yourself losing your patience constantly, consider it a wake-up call that you probably need more help. Whether the stress is coming from loss of sleep, worry, frazzled nerves, or another source, you need respite. Look into adult day programs or hiring an elder companion. See if a relative will spell you for some set number of hours a day or week.

To avoid future slips:

- If your anger is usually targeted at your loved one, remind yourself that he can't change. You have to. Try to see the situation (confusing the phone and TV remote or endless repetition) from his perspective.

- Try taking a few deep breaths at the moment you feel your fury rising. You'd be surprised how quickly it switches one kind of biological response to another. Some caregivers get to a similar place via prayer.

Tip: "When I lose it or feel myself about to, I chant to myself: 'It's okay, let it go.'" — L.G.

- More tactics when you feel the heat rising: Tackle a repetitive household chore that requires energy, like scouring pans, chopping vegetables, or mowing grass. Lift hand weights for a few reps.

- Physically remove yourself from the situation for a moment. Some people have said they excuse themselves to do a "silent scream" in the bathroom or a louder one in the car in the garage. Better yet: Practice preventative removal. Give yourself little breaks every couple of hours to have a cup of tea, look at the paper, sit outside and gaze at the sky. Caregivers need breaks, period.

- Ask yourself if there's a constructive solution to situations that make you angry repeatedly: Is compromise possible? Would being more assertive (which is different from anger) help you have a better sense of control?

- Don't try to fit three errands in a two-errand time slot. The math is against you. And make that one errand if the person with dementia is with you.

- If you notice a pattern forming, you need outlets for your pent-up feelings. Maybe more exercise, or a different kind, would help. Do you have friends you can talk to? A journal you can write in? (Even if you burn pages right after, research shows that getting the words out eases your burden.) An online caregiver chat group?

o o o

When You Grieve (Even Though Your Loved One Is Alive)

Some common scenarios:

- *Mourning what once was. Reminders of the way your loved one used to be, before Alzheimer's, can be painful when you look at old photographs or bump into your loved one's former colleagues who ask how he's doing.*

- *Mourning what is now. Your loved one is alive, and yet every day brings new sad realities. Widowed friends tell you that "at least" your loved one is still alive. Or is he? Alzheimer's isn't called "the longest goodbye" for nothing.*

- *Mourning the future that will, and won't, be. A retirement bungalow in the country that won't happen. A long-saved-for cruise that won't be shared. A father who won't give a toast at his daughter's wedding. A grandchild who won't know her grandparent.*

What you should know about grief:

The unique grief of a dementia caregiver is every bit as real and intense as the type of mourning that takes place after a death, experts say. It consists of two different psychological states experienced at once:

1. Anticipatory grief: coping with very real feelings of loss for someone who is alive

2. Ambiguous loss: interacting with someone who's not fully present socially or mentally

Alzheimer's involves a series of losses: The loss of the ability to work, to drive, to cook, to read and write, to manage basic self care, to engage fully with the world. Although we're encouraged by insightful experts to focus on what is, rather than what isn't,

294

it's impossible to completely overlook this torrent of losses. We grieve each of them.

University of Indianapolis researchers asked more than 400 caregivers the open-ended question, "What would you say is the biggest barrier you have faced as a caregiver" The majority — more than 80 percent — referred to the loss of the person they used to know.

What can help you:

- **Please believe that your feelings are normal.** It can help simply to know that anticipatory grief exists. Don't fall into the trap of thinking that because your loved one is still alive, you aren't entitled to dark emotions. Nor does it make any sense that you should be expected to hold them in.

- **Let go of associated guilt.** People often feel guilty for experiencing the difficult feelings that go along with anticipatory grief and ambiguous loss. But they're very real and logical emotions. Why wouldn't you be sad and mournful about the great changes at hand. True, your loved one is still "here," but we all know it's possible to be both here and not here, in Alzheimer's World.

- **Understand that it's "real" grief.** A 2001 study in the journal *The Gerontologist* described anticipatory grief as equivalent in intensity and breadth to the response to death. The odd silver lining: Anticipatory grief prepares us for the eventual end. It's a long, slow, painful warm-up, but it *is* a warm-up. (Not that you'll be inoculated against intense sadness and mourning later.)

- **Stay realistic about how hard dementia care is.** Many caregivers wax poetic about those unexpected "I love you's" or sudden bursts of clarity and gratitude. They're fulfilling and should be embraced, by all means. But the rest of the time — well, there's the rest of the time. Don't beat yourself up if you struggle with some aspects of caregiving.

- **Be nice to yourself.** Grief (anticipatory or otherwise) puts you at risk for depression. Depression puts *you* at risk for dementia. How to get off this vicious cycle? Start small — enlist a regular volunteer or paid aide to take over while you do something positive for your own health, such as working out. Make self-care a priority in your caregiving day; they're intimately related.

- **Rely on a support network for an emotional outlet.** You may feel the need to put on a "brave face" in front of the sick person all the time, when expressing your conflicting feelings is what would serve *you* better. A support network lets you do that. Spousal caregivers can have a tougher time getting out and connecting with friends and relatives, especially if you have health issues yourself. Yet spouses are especially at risk for depression. Venting on paper — writing about your feelings — can help during those moments when you can't see someone face to face. Long-term studies have found that Alzheimer's caregivers who receive counseling and support, formal or informal, have better health and a lower incidence of depression.

- **Consider a legacy project.** Many families are buoyed, or at least distracted, from the pain of loss by actively celebrating the life of the person with Alzheimer's. Sample projects include recording an audiovisual life story (in the mild to moderate stages), pulling together a scrapbook or photo album, writing a biography, or organizing and documenting a collection or other endeavor representative of your loved one's life. It doesn't have to be a life record. A legacy project can also be the creation of something your loved one leaves behind — a joke book for grandchildren, lap robes knit for charity, marching in an Alzheimer's walk.

In some cases, it's a project you can focus on together — transforming feelings of pain into pride and meaning. A legacy project is also a terrific distraction that helps you feel productive.

- **Explore hospice.** Eventually, the person in your care will descend into end-stage Alzheimer's (or succumb to another illness first). Finding out about hospice programs near you, and what they entail, isn't a secret death wish, as some people mistakenly believe. You can't control the timing of the end. But it does come, and you deserve the skilled guidance that experts in this passage can offer you, even if it's still months (or more) in the unknowable future.

o o o

PRACTICAL STRESSORS

Lack of Privacy

Some common scenarios:

- *Not the Waltons:* Even TV's Appalachia-poor Waltons family had an old farmhouse bigger than your suburban split-level. Night after night, everyone sits in the cramped family room arguing over what to watch on TV. At dinner, the conversation is tense and strained as Grandpa struggles to get the food in his mouth and the kids can't wait to snarf and split.

- *Not the Golden Girls:* Your parent moved in — and now expects to do everything with you. Or your spouse has become overly clingy, following you everywhere.

- *Not the stuff of home movies, either:* Your mom thinks nothing of walking into your bedroom, even when the door is shut. Dad rifles through the papers on your desk while you're at work, and you can't find anything. When you go to the bathroom, your grandmother knocks — every time — asking, "Are you in there? Is anybody in there?"

What you should know about privacy:

Everyone in a caregiving family needs the freedom to exist in his or her own space. Having physical privacy means having boundaries that let everyone in the household escape 24/7 interactions. This is especially challenging in small living spaces.

And with dementia, it's easy for even loving families to feel way too close for comfort. Your loved one may need help with basic needs, from meal planning to toileting. Disinhibition (loss of social appropriateness) may lead your loved one to barge into bedrooms and bathrooms. Or you may be shadowed closely wherever you go.

It's not just your sanity at stake. You also need the privacy to be able to continue with some version of long-established family time and traditions. Ideally, you weave your live-in family member into family life, while balancing the need for kids and spouses to have their own routines and share of your attention.

What can help you:

- **Create to-each-his-own spaces.** If you can afford it, make home improvements to allow your live-in elder to have his or her own living quarters, not just for sleeping but also for living: a TV set and comfortable chair, a desk, even (in a perfect world) a small refrigerator or kitchenette. Separate living and sleeping quarters are ideal so that only rest and sleep happen in the bedroom, minimizing sleep problems.

- Explore whether a parent's assets can be used to fund a modest addition to your home. This is often a cheaper alternative to out-of-home care and can increase the value of the home

- **Preserve non-elder time.** Remain conscious of maintaining one-on-one time with other family members. Your live-in parent doesn't always have to come first with you; use respite care or other relatives to supplement care

- **Get physically away.** Everyone in the house needs opportunities to get away, especially a hands-on caregiver. Don't put vacations, school or sports events, or other previous family activities on indefinite hold

- **Don't be afraid to use locks.** When someone with dementia begins to invade your private space, logic and kind requests will do little good. Install simple deadbolts in your bedroom and master bath. (You'll still get interrupted but without the intrusion.)

  Locks in bathrooms are trickier because you don't want the person to accidentally lock himself in and be unable to get out. Experts often recommend to removing bathroom locks for this reason. One option: locks that can be opened from either side. These may be tricky

299

enough to keep your loved one out but still allow you to go in, if needed. Plastic doorknob covers that are hard to grip can also deter someone from entering rooms.

- **Remember that kids need space, too.** Avoid making a child share a room with an elder if you can. While family togetherness is nice, don't force caregiving responsibilities. It's fair to expect any child to respect an elder and for an older child or teen to help some with care tasks, but take care to preserve their independence and childhood. It doesn't help anyone if a child nurses resentment.

- **If boundary-intruding becomes overwhelming:** Mention these behaviors to the doctor, especially if they take a sudden change for the more insistent. Medication interactions or alcohol use can worsen behaviors, or there may be another underlying cause. Eventually, for your own health and your loved one's safety, you may not be able to live under one roof.

o o o

Lack of "Me" Time

Some common scenarios:

- *Feeling like a hermit. You used to have a social life. You went to book club, met people for dinner or the odd dishy lunch. You got your hair done, instead of pulling it back into an ever-longer ponytail. Now, you can't even remember when you got out to the mall, just meandering around at your own pace.*

- *Feeling unfit. You hear about the importance of exercise and self care over and over, but who has time to get to the gym? Heck, who has time — since you can't leave your loved one home alone — to walk around the block? And if you bring her with you, it means getting all the aerobic output of a snail.*

- *Feeling like a stranger to yourself. There's no time for reading a Twitter feed, much less the latest novel. You shower instead of luxuriate in the bath. Some days, you feel you can barely hear yourself think. Your own thoughts don't seem to matter, anyway, crowded out as they are by worries, doctor appointments, medication reminders, toileting reminders, drink-more-water-Dad reminders.*

What you should know about taking time for yourself:

Though everyone values the idea of "me" time, many caregivers are convinced they can't find any. It's not easy, but it's always possible. Start small, dream big.

You'll be better able to weather stress. Have more energy. Think more clearly. Feel less overwhelmed. Better avert depression. Be healthier and able to provide better care, longer.

What can help you:

- **Yes, start small:** Aim for just 10 or 15 minutes daily if you feel it's hopeless. Literally write what you'll do on your planner or daily to-do list. Commit to carving this same time out every day. (Don't plan to randomly grab 15 minutes whenever you can.) Life coaches say it can take up to three weeks for a new habit to take hold. Devoting specific times to yourself helps you make "me" time a priority. What can you do in just 10 or 15 minutes that will make a difference? Pump free weights (start with two- or three-pound dumbbells). Write a letter to someone or keep a diary. Make a playlist of your favorite high-energy or sing-along tunes and crank them up. Music with a strong beat is known to boost energy; orchestral and acoustic music can improve thinking.

- **Schedule time for yourself early in your day.** Don't make personal time an afterthought or reward *after* you finish the day's business. Mark out "you" time early in the day, so the day doesn't run away on you. Plus, you'll be better able to face the day if you're more energized.

- **Make the break feel like an indulgence.** No laundry. No paying the bills. Think of something you enjoyed when you had more time, before your life got crazy. Maybe it's savoring a cup of tea in a china cup while reading a brand-new book you've downloaded. Or setting up a craft table to pursue an art or project you've abandoned.

- **Now go broader:** After a week or so of adding a daily break, block out a larger span of time at least weekly to do something self-indulgent away from home. Get a massage or a manicure, wander the mall, attend a book group.

Tip: "I make time for prayer every morning. It's something I've always done, but now I treasure the time more than ever — to ask for strength and then feel calm and ready for anything after. I think meditation or yoga or whatever your source of spiritual strength is would do the same if you do it early and every day." — E.F.

- **Just say "No."** If you're tempted to yield to a request, get in the habit of replying, "I'm not sure; let me get back to you." Even if you're pretty sure you're able to do it, don't answer immediately. Give yourself a cushion of time to reflect privately on whether the request will enhance your life or detract from it. Saying "no" is like working a muscle. The more you express regrets or bow out, the easier it becomes the next time.

If you find it hard to refuse others (and this is true for many people with caregiver hearts), rehearse a few lines to fall back on: "I'd love to help, but I just have too much going on right now." Or, "I wish I could, but it will have to be another time." Humor helps: "If I take on even one more thing, my husband will divorce me and my hair will catch on fire." Be especially protective if indulging a favor or taking on a new task would nip into your personal time. You'll never find enough time for yourself if you don't cordon it off.

- **Create a "you" cave.** It could be a whole spare bedroom or a desk and comfy chair in a corner. Decorate your "me zone" with meaningful mementos, a comfy quilt, your favorite photos.

Having your own personal retreat ensures you'll be more likely to head there to do something just for yourself — watch a DVD, Skype with an old high school pal, run through some yoga moves, take a power nap. Ask others in the house to respect your privacy when you're in your personal space. (It doesn't always work, but it never hurts to ask!)

- **Try a portable "you" zone.** When you can't get to your special space and you're feeling overwhelmed, remember that you can clear a "me zone" in your head. Close your eyes and take a few calming deep breaths. (Some people find it helpful to retreat to the bathroom to get this kind of privacy.) Or do a "mind sweep": Jot down all the things troubling you (conflicts, to-do items). The simple act of making a list releases some of the tension and helps you prioritize.

- **Share your load.** Spend less time on things that don't absolutely require your personal involvement by delegating, rotating, or outsourcing. For most families, even when one person is the primary caregiver, giving care is a family-wide experience. Is there anyone in your household who can make dinner one night a week? Run a vacuum? Cut the lawn? Enlist kids as well as adults. Perhaps one person could clean up as you cook, reducing the need for a big clean after. Post a chore schedule, with everybody taking a shift. Look into sharing the marketing or a carpool with a neighbor. Consider a "parent-sitting" exchange with a friend who also has a live-in elderly parent who can't stay alone.

- **Don't discount the person with dementia as a helper.** Don't do things for older relatives that they can still do for themselves. Too often, caregivers err on the side of "helping" to excess. Until late-stage Alzheimer's, activities such as cleaning or folding laundry can provide an elder with a healthful sense of usefulness and contribution.

  It's fine to work side-by-side if your loved one wouldn't be safe working alone. But resist the urge to help, hover, or take over because the job isn't meeting your standards. Figure out which things you can let go.

- **Look for shortcuts and other streamlining efficiencies.** For one whole day, analyze the way you do all your routine tasks with an eye toward saving time. For example, paying bills online is faster than writing checks, stuffing envelopes, scrambling for stamps, and mailing them. It's a tiny time difference, but the saved minutes add up.

  Could you make lunches every other day, preparing two at a time? Or make a casserole or pot of soup you can heat up for several days running? Plan errands for times of day when crowds are thinner (avoiding lunchtime and rush hour, for example). Scheduling morning medical appointments, or the first appointment after lunch, means less waiting-room time, because the doctor is less likely to have gotten backed up.

- **Tackle the dregs first.** Try to get your least favorite or hardest tasks out of the way early in the day, when you have more energy. That way you'll chip through more pleasant jobs during the rest of the day with a sense of accomplishment, rather than energy-draining dread.

  Or double up: Pair a task you don't like with one you do. Iron or run on the treadmill while you catch up on a prerecorded favorite TV show or reach out to a friend by cell phone to chat (and vent as needed!). If you're paying bills online, open up a second window to chat with fellow caregivers in an online forum. Invest in an electronic reader (like the Kindle or iPad) to download new books or magazines without having to take the time to go to the library or bookstore. And you'll always have escapist reading material at your fingertips in doctors' waiting rooms, on the bus, in between errands.

- **Take mini-breaks.** We all need more escapes than we can get in a day or week. Try an occasional quick-fix throughout your day. Paced deep breathing is known to lower heart rate and blood pressure. Or treat yourself to a square of dark chocolate. Yes, it can actually lower stress hormones, according to a 2009 Swiss (where else?) study, which gave people a two-inch square every day for two weeks — half was eaten at mid-morning and half at midafternoon. (But don't beat yourself up if you can't make it last that long.)

  A neat de-stressing trick: Relive a "memory photo." The next time you're having a wonderful experience — a birthday party, a quiet walk by yourself in a beautiful place, a simple interaction with your loved one — take a "memory snapshot." Imprint the memory on your mind by focusing intently on everything you can about the moment, using all of your senses. What do you see up close and all around you? Take in the colors, the textures, the details. What does it smell like? What does a kiss or piece of chocolate cake taste like? Spending just 30 seconds consciously taking in as much as you can about a moment helps imprint it on your brain, making the full experience easier to recall later. Then, when you're stressed, close your eyes and conjure up the memory you "photographed." It's a quickie escape that can recapture the positive feelings you had in that moment — and bring them into your present.

- **Unplug.** As much as electronic gadgets help us multitask, they can also become time-suckers that lead us to squander downtime moments we didn't realize we hand. That's how we wind up zoning in front of the TV all evening (watching something we don't even like) or flipping through catalogs and Reddit for hours and yet never feeling like we have time to ourselves.

  Try starting with 15 "silent" minutes a day — if it plugs in, unplug it or turn it off. You don't necessarily have to spend that time on yourself to feel like you've gained something. The quality of your interactions with others will seem deeper when you focus more on one another. And your psyche comes away refreshed without the chronic distraction of competing interests.

- **Buy time.** Don't underestimate the value of outsourcing. Yes, it means spending money. But your time carries a price tag, too — and your health and peace of mind are priceless. Weigh the costs of a biweekly cleaning service against the time you spend on such tasks now. Look into a grocery delivery service or take-out meals, which many supermarkets now offer. Pay a neighborhood kid to handle yard work and to clean gutters. Hire a teenager to relieve you every afternoon at five for an hour, so you can take an exercise class. (Ask a local Scout troop or high school for reliable candidates.) A free option: local church youth groups or schools, which often require students to earn service hours by helping those in need.

Professional caregivers, from nurse aides to elder companions, can help in the home. Adult day programs, for those able to attend them, are another source of "found hours" for you and a win-win, since most people are energized by attending them. Resist the excuse that nobody can care as well as you can. That may well be true, but many paid professionals do a darn good job — and when your sanity is at stake, that's plenty good .

- **Don't be shy about asking for the gift of time.** If your budget is stretched, consider asking relatives who have offered to help if they'll pay for specific kinds of relief. Many of us hate to "talk money," but long distance caregivers who can't give their time often welcome such an opportunity to feel like they're making a difference. And when someone asks what you (or your loved one) want for your birthday or a holiday, ask for the gift of time (or the money to buy it).

  The trick is to apply the time you buy toward *yourself*, not anything or anyone else. If an aide or a sibling spends time with your loved one on Saturday mornings, go out to do something personally meaningful during that block of time — don't just run errands. By having short breaks from each other, you and your loved one will both be more apt to come together again stimulated by the change and — critical for you — renewed.

- **Don't discount the person with dementia as a helper.** Don't do things for older relatives that they can still do for themselves. Too often, caregivers err on the side of "helping" to excess. Until late-stage Alzheimer's, activities such as cleaning or folding laundry can provide an elder with a healthful sense of usefulness and contribution. It's fine to work side-by-side if your loved one wouldn't be safe working alone. But resist the urge to help, hover, or take over because the job isn't meeting your standards. Figure out which things you can let go.

o o o

Your Sleep Problems (Insomnia, Sleep Deprivation)

Some common scenarios:

- *Kept awake by worry. Whether the topic is money, care logistics, or any of 1,000 other concerns on your plate, ruminating in the dark is a sure path to insomnia.*

- *Disrupted by Alzheimer's. If your loved one keeps getting up to use the bathroom or pace the halls, chances are your sleep cycle will be disrupted, too. When day and night are completely mixed up due to dementia, the whole household can suffer.*

- *Burning the candle at both ends. There are only so many hours to do soooooo many things. Many caregivers rise extra early and stay up extra late. The house is often quiet, but this "found time" is stolen from sleep.*

- *Body gone haywire. Caregivers tend to be mid-lifers or older, ages when our own bodies experience problems that can disrupt sleep, separate from our loved one's Alzheimer's or from caregiving itself. On this list: Menopause, bladder problems, prostate problems, thyroid disorders, restless leg syndrome, sleep apnea, and medication interactions, to name a few.*

What you should know about sleep problems:

Sleep scientists now know well that getting enough sleep, and of good quality, is a linchpin to overall health and stress levels. Sleep is protective against disorders ranging from obesity to heart disease. Sleep boosts mood. Sleep gives energy. Sleep helps us organize our memories and protects brain function. Far from being useless downtime into which you should cram laundry, paperwork, and computer surfing, night hours should be your best friend in your quest to provide good quality care for as long as possible.

In short, you can't get along very well, or go very far, without sleep.

For all these reasons, getting sufficient sleep makes you a better caregiver. The irony is that caregivers often ignore their own disturbed or insufficient sleep because it just doesn't seem as critical as all the other fires that need putting out in a day. Or it may feel like an insurmountable problem.

What can help you:

In general:

- **Know that if dementia-disrupted sleep is the root cause, you must address it.** Caregivers too often excuse or ignore sleep problems in the person they look after. There are two main reasons, says geriatric psychiatrist Ken Robbins. First, they mistakenly assume that poor sleep is just part of aging, or part of dementia, and think nothing can be done about it. Second, they fear that making a big issue about it and seeking medical help is just a selfish act — as if the sleep problem were only theirs, and not a shared one. Solving sleep problems helps everyone.

- **Be honest about other symptoms.** Along with feeling tired and draggy, do you notice other physical changes that you've been ignoring? A racing pulse? Feeling out of breath on stairs? A leaky bladder when you laugh or sneeze? Sleep may be related to another health issue you should have checked out now by your doctor. Don't just complain about the sleep — take inventory of anything else bothering you, and report it.

Also be aware that waking up tired even after you think you've slept is one of the warning signs of sleep apnea, a common (and fortunately treatable) condition that causes people to miss breaths while they sleep.

Before going to bed:

- **Get the basics down.** You may not be able to control when you're awakened, but at least you can structure an environment that's pro-sleep when you're there. These are the same tips as for someone with dementia who awakens: The bedroom should be cool, quiet, and dark. Take out the TV; don't play the radio or use a laptop there. Change into sleep attire — even if you prefer sweats or lounge PJ's, make these items you wear only for bed, not for daytime, too.

- **Try over-the-counter sleep aids for a few nights.** They can help you restore your sleep cycle and get needed rest. But don't use them more than a few nights a week for more than a few weeks — that's a sign you should have yourself checked out. The doctor may also be able to prescribe a stronger sleep medicine. Some caregivers swear by melatonin, a hormone sold at drugstores.

- **Pick the right nightcap.** Alcohol? No — it will help you nod off but then awaken you later as it moves through your system. Warm milk — yes. The amino acid it contains really does help to calm you. Avoid caffeine crutches (coffee, tea, cocoa) after early afternoon.

- **Eat for sleep.** Oatmeal before bed can elevate your blood sugar in a way that triggers sleep-inducing brain chemicals and keeps blood sugar steady, so you can sleep. Oats also contain vitamin B6 and melatonin, which promote relaxation. Bananas are another source of melatonin, as well as serotonin. Go for the sleep-lulling trifecta: oatmeal made with milk and topped with banana.

- **Think calming down, not revving up.** If you're having sleep trouble, avoid exercising at night. Instead try gentle stretching, meditation, yoga, or relaxation moves. A good example of the latter: Systematically clench and release each major muscle group, starting at your forehead and moving down to your toes. Avoid scheduling family conference calls or updates to relatives late in the day before bed if these conversations risk riling you up.

When you wake up at night:

- **Don't blend day and night yourself.** When you do get up at night, keep the room dark. Leave the room to read, watch TV, or tend to your loved one. Try to keep sleep space and activities separate from waking ones.

  One trick that helps ruminators who can't stop their thoughts from racing: Keep a notebook on your bedside table. Write down what you're thinking about. Committing the worrisome thoughts — or a possible To Do list — to paper can help you jettison it from your brain for a while, so you can rest.

- **Repeat the evening relaxers:** Have a glass of warm milk. Do progressive relaxation exercises. Avoid electronics.

More help:

- **Practice the power nap.** The good news about naps is that they're linked to lower blood pressure, less heart disease, healthy weight, more energy, and improved mood — the same benefits as nighttime sleep. An oft-quoted study in the journal *Sleep* pinpointed the ideal nap length at 10 minutes. Sleep more than 30 minutes and you start to cycle into sleep stages that mean you'll wake up feeling groggy, not refreshed.

  One trick: The caffeine nap. Have a cup of coffee about 20 minutes before a short nap. It takes about half an hour for caffeine to kick in. So shortly after you wake up, the java will jolt, leaving you doubly energized.

- **Consider p.m. respite care.** If you absolutely need to sleep at night, try hiring a night nurse or aide to be on duty at least a few nights a week. Even if your loved one doesn't always get up at night, just knowing that someone else is in charge for a few hours can provide the peace of mind you need to fall into deep and restorative slumber.

o o o

"Don't feel bad about asking for help. Caring is a team sport!"

— *Ira Byock, MD, author of* The Best Care Possible

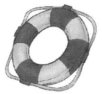

4 RESOURCES

A toolkit for family caregivers

Here, you'll find:

Stages of Alzheimer's: Overview

- **How it can help:** It will give you know where you are and what's ahead, so can you can gird yourself and plan.

Test Yourself: Are You Headed for Burnout?

- **How it can help:** Like the proverbial frog in heating water, we often don't realize we're being boiled alive by slow-but-relentless stress. Use this quiz as an early-warning system for your own health and well being.

11 Warning Signs of Depression

- **How it can help:** Both people with dementia and their live-in help are at raised risk for this life-changer —use it to stop wondering and know exactly what to look for.

More Sources of Help

- **How it can help:** These are the resources every dementia caregiver should know. Use them to find respite care, dementia education, clinical trials, medication information, local meals or transportation services, kindred spirits, and more.

o o o

Stages of Alzheimer's: Overview

You might be surprised to learn that there's no single definition of the "stages of Alzheimer's." Several different staging approaches are used. They all reflect the fact that Alzheimer's is a progressive disease (it gets gradually worse) along a spectrum.

Please remember that "Alzheimer's" is a form of dementia. Dementia refers to a collection of behaviors and symptoms that interfere with daily life. There are many different causes of dementia, such as stroke, Lewy Body disease, Parkinson's, and alcoholism. Alzheimer's is just one kind of dementia, by far the most common cause. With some exceptions, the progression of decline with dementia tends to be the same, whatever the cause.

Because you might encounter any of the three following ways of staging Alzheimer's dementia, I'm including all of them. The most useful to caregivers, I think, because of its practicality and ease of understanding, is the third one. It's also fairly applicable to dementia of any type.

1. Diagnostic guidelines for Alzheimer's dementia and MCI

The newest way to classify Alzheimer's disease was defined in spring, 2011, following a two-year congress of leading researchers, sponsored by the National Institute on Aging and the Alzheimer's Association. Its stages are as follows:

- *Preclinical Alzheimer's*, also called pre-symptomatic: This newest stage, first defined in 2011, is when changes are seen in the brain and blood (now that such biomarkers can be seen through brain imaging and other tests) but the person doesn't show behavioral or cognitive symptoms. This stage is currently of greatest value to researchers.

- *Mild cognitive impairment (MCI) due to Alzheimer's*: Mild changes in memory and thinking ability are noticeable to the person and to family and friends but don't interfere with the ability to carry out daily activities. Most, but not all, cases of MCI eventually develop into Alzheimer's.

- *Dementia due to Alzheimer's.* This is the stage most people think of as "Alzheimer's": Memory, thinking, and behavioral symptoms increasingly impair the person's ability to function in everyday life.

2. Seven stages of Alzheimer's

Developed by Dr. Barry Reisberg and popularized by the Alzheimer's Association, this "global deterioration scale" is a complex listing that's still often referred to:

- *Stage 1:* No impairment; a normal person

- *Stage 2:* Very mild cognitive decline that may or may not be normal aging

- *Stage 3:* Mild cognitive decline: Memory problems obvious to others

- *Stage 4:* Moderate cognitive decline: Mild-stage Alzheimer's

- *Stage 5:* Moderately severe cognitive decline: Moderate or mid-stage Alzheimer's

- *Stage 6:* Severe cognitive decline: Moderately severe or mid-stage Alzheimer's

- *Stage 7:* Very severe cognitive decline: Severe or late-stage Alzheimer's

3. Mild-moderate-severe dementia staging

Probably the most widely used staging system due to its ease of

316

use, this approach refers to three main stages of dementia: mild, moderate and severe. Because they chart a progression, they're sometimes further subdivided (early mild, mid-mild, late mild, early moderate, and so on).

Mild stage Alzheimer's: The person can still manage basic self care and communicate well, but memory changes are interfering with the so-called "instrumental activities of daily living" (IADLs), the higher-order thinking skills that one gains in the teenage years, such as driving, preparing meals, and managing money. Someone with mild-stage Alzheimer's may:

- Repeat questions and comments

- Misuse words

- Get lost on familiar routes

- Seem preoccupied or irritable, or show other personality changes

- Have trouble with basic finances, transportation, and medications.

The earliest mild-stage Alzheimer's overlaps with mild cognitive impairment, the stage when the cause of such changes still seems unclear. But with Alzheimer's-type dementia, problems continue to increase.

Moderate-stage Alzheimer's: The person begins to have trouble with the so-called "activities of daily living" (ADLs), which are basic skills gained during childhood, such as grooming, feeding, and toileting. Someone with moderate-stage Alzheimer's may:

- Fidget restlessly, pace, wander away from home, get lost

- Experience evening agitation known as sundowning

- Remember the distant past better than recent events

- Need help choosing clothes or dressing, getting to the toilet, or bathing.

Severe-stage Alzheimer's: The person becomes unable to perform the activities of daily living without significant help. Basic life skills such as those gained during the first year of life (speaking, walking, continence) are also affected. Someone with severe-stage Alzheimer's may:

- Seem to lose all memory and live in a constant present

- Be unable to talk intelligibly

- Not recognize even close family

- Lose the ability to walk or sit up unassisted.

Because people with Alzheimer's tend to have bad days and good days, it can sometimes be hard to tell where in the progression they are. If you look at the big picture, though, you see a generally increasing decline. The length of each stage varies widely by individual. There's no one template for this disease. A person can seem to pass quickly through a stage, or stay in it for years. The final stage is typically longest, according to the Alzheimer's Association's 2013 report, Alzheimer's Disease Facts and Figures.

What is the overall life expectancy with Alzheimer's? Someone diagnosed at 85 or later typically lives for several years after diagnosis; those who are younger at diagnosis tend to live longer. The Alzheimer's Association report says that among those 65 or older, average survival from diagnosis to death is four to eight years; rarely, people survive for up to 20 years. Of course, older adults tend to have other chronic diseases on top of dementia and may actually die from a different cause.

o o o

Test Yourself: Are You Headed for Burnout?

"Caregiving requires a certain amount of selflessness, but it's important for caregivers to know their limits. Caregivers can become so focused on the person they're assisting that they neglect their own needs."

— *geriatric psychiatrist Ken Robbins*

Caregiving can bring many positives into your life — but it's also hard work for your your body, mind, and soul. Without enough self-care to replenish your reserves, stresses of all kinds can build.

Before you know it, they can reach the toxic levels of caregiver burnout, a syndrome of mental, emotional, and physical depletion. When you're burned out, you have a hard time being responsive and providing the level of care you'd like. Burnout also raises your risk of chronic depression and other mental and physical ailments, from hypertension and flu to diabetes and stroke — or even premature death. Caregiver burnout is also a leading cause of nursing home placement, when run-down caregivers become too depleted to manage caregiving demands.

What's *your* caregiver burnout index? Answer the following 12 questions.

1. How often do you get a good night's sleep (seven or more hours)?

a. Every night

b. Most nights

c. A few times a week

d. Seldom or never

2. How often do you keep up with leisure activities that you enjoyed before caregiving?

a. Every day

b. Often

c. Sometimes

d. Seldom or never

3. How often do you feel irritable or lose your temper with your loved one or others?

a. Seldom or never

b. Sometimes

c. Often

d. Every day

4. How often do you feel happy?

a. Every day

b. Often

c. Sometimes

d. Seldom or never

5. How often do you find it difficult to concentrate?

a. Seldom or never

b. Sometimes

c. Often

d. Every day

6. How often do you need a cigarette, more than two cups of coffee, junk foods, or a similar substance crutch to make it through the day?

a. Seldom or never

b. Sometimes

c. Often

d. Every day

7. How often do you lack the energy to cook, clean, and take care of everyday basics?

a. Seldom or never

b. Sometimes

c. Often

d. Every day

8. How often do you feel hopeless about the future?

a. Seldom or never

b. Sometimes

c. Often

d. Every day

9. How often are you able to relax without the use of alcohol or prescription sedatives?

a. Every day

b. Often

c. Sometimes

d. Seldom or never

10. How often do you feel utterly overwhelmed by all you have to do?

a. Seldom or never

b. Sometimes

c. Often

d. Every day

11. How often has someone criticized your caregiving or suggested you're burning out?

a. Seldom or never

b. Sometimes

c. Often

d. Every day

12. How often do you feel that someone is looking after or caring for *you*?

a. Every day

b. Often

c. Sometimes

d. Seldom or never

How did you score?

This self-test isn't a scientific or diagnostic measure; it's meant to help you identify whether your stress level warrants taking steps toward better protecting yourself.

Add up your score. Each A = 4 points, B = 3 points, C = 2 points, D = 1 point.

What your score means:

48-42: Good, you're keeping your cool (low burnout risk)

Your heart and head are both in the right place, and your stress-busting reservoirs are full, which helps you give care with grace and good humor. That said, caregiver stress often creeps up without a caregiver realizing it. Protecting your healthful habits is paramount.

What to do: Keep yourself well fueled for caring by making time for yourself every day — at minimum, aim for several five-minute pick-me-ups for caregiver stress. If you're in a relationship, know that a healthy marriage or other close relationship where you can vent and feel appreciated is a good source of strength.

30-41: Be careful, you're feverish (elevated burnout risk)

You're likely managing caregiver stress reasonably well but falling into a common trap: letting yourself sink lower on the daily priority list than is optimal. Everyone has an occasional crazy-busy day, but too many of such days brings chronic stress. That's what erodes well-being and places you at risk for depression, colds, and other illnesses.

What to do: Protect your time for self-care, even if it's just grabbing short pick-me-ups: a chapter a day of a good novel, awakening early for a walk before your loved one is up, a twice-a-week meet-up with a friend. It might seem inconsequential to focus on eating more healthy foods or lifting hand weights, but small steps can make a big change in your overall health — and ultimately, in your ability to provide better care.

18-29: Your life may be too hot to handle (high burnout risk)

Your stress level is probably sky-high. You may already be experiencing dangerous symptoms of anxiety, depression, compromised immunity, and physical exhaustion. It's critical that you take steps immediately to lower your stress level, ideally through a combination of better self-care, a shared workload, and outlets for your complicated emotions, including talk therapy and support groups.

What to do: In addition to the suggestions in the sections above, know the 11 warning signs of depression below. A physical exam can help you uncover and treat the ill effects of stress that you might already be experiencing. Having an outlet for someone to talk to can also ease your burden.

One of the best strategies for managing fireballing burnout is respite care. Check into community resources as well as your network of supporters to find ways to ease your 24/7 burden. It's never too early to look into alternate housing plans, as difficult as that may be. It can be lifesaving.

12-17: Feeling like toast? (you might already be burned out)

It's a wonder — and a blessing — that you were able to take this quiz. You're running on empty, or perhaps barely running at all. Although you want to do your best for the person you're caring for, realize that your own health is at stake — and if you don't look out for yourself now, you won't be able to help the person or persons in your care.

What to do: You need immediate help. Learn how to tell the difference between the normal stress of caregiving and depression and consult with someone you trust — a doctor, clergyperson, counselor, or therapist for counseling — and seek out medical assistance. At minimum, you need a physical checkup. You may also benefit from other therapies or from a break from caregiving that's as short-term as a vacation or as permanent as a relocation of the person in your care. Many caregivers find that when care tasks become overwhelming —

and there are many reasons why this happens — they're able to show more love and support by not being a hands-on caregiver. That results in everyone being healthier and happier, including the person with dementia.

o o o

11 *Warning Signs of Depression*

If you're a caregiver, it's important to understand depression. It's not just a bad or sad mood; it's a physical disease that can affect both your loved one and you.

You're both at elevated risk. Almost half of those with Alzheimer's become clinically depressed, so some of the changes you write off to the disease may actually be reversible because they're caused by the depression, which is treatable. What's more, caregivers develop dementia at twice the rate of non-caregivers. Spousal caregivers are at highest risk. Depression can make it challenging, or even impossible, to continue providing care.

True clinical depression differs from the blues in two key ways:

- Severity: Symptoms are difficult enough to deal with that they interfere with everyday life.

- Duration: Symptoms are present nearly all the time and last for more than two weeks.

The following 11 warning signs indicate that someone isn't dealing with normal, temporary emotions but instead with the illness of depression. Symptoms vary by individual: A depressed person isn't likely to have all 11 symptoms at once, and their severity may shift. Depression can be mild or major; either way, if several symptoms are present and last for more than two weeks, you or someone you're concerned about may need medical help.

1. Persistent sad, anxious, or "empty" feelings

This symptom looks like a low mood but persists even after time goes by and the cause of the bad mood has cleared up or receded.

What to look for: Blank stares, loss of interest in life, an inability to feel or express happiness or other emotions. Or the person may report just feeling "empty" or "numb."

What else to know: Often the depressed person isn't fully aware of this symptom. Try asking, "When's the last time you were happy?"

2. Feelings of hopelessness, worthlessness, or helplessness

In an "Eeyore-like" pessimistic way, the depressed person can't help feeling that everything is wrong and it's his or her fault (rather than the fault of the situation or the illness itself). It's a hallmark sign of major depression. In mild depression, the feelings are similar but less extreme.

How to tell: The person seems unable to see any positive flip side to things or light at the end of the tunnel — and feels little sense of control over choices or events. The person talks and acts as if he or she has no options, can't see a different path, is useless and meaningless. He or she may fixate on past mistakes, ruminating over them and expressing guilt and self blame.

What else to know: Listen for comments like these: "It's hopeless." "I can't do anything about it." "I have no choice." "Nobody cares." "I'm stuck." "I should have/could have/ if only...."

3. Frequent crying episodes

The crying may not seem to have a direct or obvious trigger; sobs often come "out of nowhere." But it's not normal to cry every day (though the depressed person may not realize this).

What to look for: In between episodes you witness, you may notice red eyes, sniffles, cracking voice, balled-up tissues, and other trails to tears.

What else to know: Not every depressed person cries; in fact, some never do. Research has shown that women are more inclined to this behavior than men. A 2001 University of California, San Francisco study found that crying isn't related to the severity of depression and that people who cry more may have briefer depressive episodes. Also, people with advanced Alzheimer's sometimes wail and have crying jags, a form of communication that may or may not be related to mood.

4. Increased agitation and restlessness

Some people with depression fall on the "hyper" end of a spectrum of behaviors, while others are the opposite (see symptom #5).

What to look for: The person may seem unable to relax, be more irritable than usual or quicker to anger, full of restless energy, seldom calm. Look for pacing, lashing out at others, frequent standing up and sitting back down.

What else to know: For the depressed person, everything seems magnified. So small slights or irritations aren't just pebbles in the psyche, they're giant boulders that get in the way of ordinary life.

5. Fatigue and decreased energy

Typically depressed people who don't show a lot of agitation and restlessness (symptom #4) experience the flip side of those behaviors — an increased sluggishness and slowness.

What to look for: The person may complain of having no energy, of feeling unproductive, or of "slowing down." He or she may have quit exercising, seem tired a lot, move more slowly, and have slowed reactions. "To-Do" lists never get finished the way they once did. The person may skip work; a caregiver may be less attentive to the person with Alzheimer's.

What else to know: Fatigue is a real mind-body problem. Low mood and loss of motivation are partly at work, as well as a physiological depletion of energy — and the two forces keep reinforcing each other.

6. Loss of interest in activities or hobbies that were once pleasurable

This is one of the single most telling symptoms of depression.

What to look for: The person no longer takes pleasure in things that once brought enjoyment, whether the lives of children or grandchildren, a hobby or craft, exercise, cooking, book club, watching sports — anything. Caregiving itself can become all-consuming, but someone who is depressed won't even find joy in brief encounters with family or friends. He or she may begin to decline invitations, refuse to go out, not want to see friends or family. This also can be seen in someone with mild dementia or mild cognitive impairment.

What else to know: Some depressed people lose interest in sex. For others, sex functions as a kind of escape, used the same way some depressed people turn to alcohol or drugs.

7. Difficulty concentrating, remembering details, and making decisions

"Fuzzy thinking" is often apparent both to the depressed person and his or her family, friends, and colleagues.

How to tell: Various mental slips may become obvious, such as forgetting appointments and errands, making checkbook errors, misplacing objects, forgetting names, avoiding making plans, postponing decisions or deferring them to others. The person may begin writing reminders to himself or herself or take a long time reading (because it's harder to focus). It may become harder to perform complicated tasks.

What else to know: Cognitive changes associated with depression can look like dementia, of course. The symptoms can indicate one problem or the other — or both simultaneously.

8. Sleeping too much or not enough

Disordered sleep and depression are closely related. In some people, depression manifests as insomnia (inability to fall sleep or to stay asleep). Others experience the opposite extreme: All the person feels like doing is sleeping.

What to look for: Regular sleep routines are disrupted; staying up too late or going to bed unusually early; being unable to awaken on time; complaining about a poor night's sleep; sleeping long hours but fitfully — so the person never feels rested; excessive napping by day.

What else to know: Depression is a leading cause of sleep problems, in part because it interferes with natural biological rhythms. Sundowning is linked to depression.

9. Poor appetite or overeating

Again, the symptom tends to show up as one extreme or the other: The person loses interest in eating or falls into a pattern of constant, emotionally triggered eating.

What to look for: Missed meals, picking at food (especially if this is a change for the person), lying about food intake; loss of interest even in formerly favorite foods, mindless munching and other mindless eating, throwing up after eating; weight gain or weight loss.

What else to know: Depression is a common cause of the eating disorders anorexia, bulimia, and binge eating. It's true both that depression can lead to eating disorders and that people with eating disorders can develop depression. Dementia itself can also disrupt eating patterns.

10. Expressing thoughts of dying or suicide

Depression is one of the conditions most commonly associated with suicide. It begins to seem like a logical way to end the pain and suffering. As many as 90 percent of those who commit suicide are clinically depressed, have a substance abuse problem, or both, according to the National Institutes of Mental Health. (Many people with depression self-medicate with alcohol, which lowers inhibitions and increases the risk for suicide.)

What to look for: The intention may be expressed directly, such as, "I wish I were dead" or "I want to kill myself," or "I want to end it all." Or the threats may be indirect: "You'd be better off without me." "I can't go on." "I wish it were over." "Soon I won't be around any more." Also beware of a preoccupation with death or evidence of plans to follow-through, like buying a gun, hoarding pills, giving away money, or suddenly changing a will.

What else to know: If you think someone you love may be suicidal, don't leave him or her alone. Rather than leaping right to asking, "Are you thinking about suicide?" ask a series of questions that build on one another to assess the person's state of mind: "How are you feeling? Are you feeling depressed? Are you feeling hopeless? Are you wondering if life is worth living? Are you considering suicide? Have you made a plan?" Encouraging the person to talk about the intended suicide actually lowers (but doesn't remove) the risk of following through. Keep the person safe until he or she can be brought to a doctor or therapist. Or call 911 or a suicide hotline. The National Suicide Prevention Lifeline is (800) 273-8255.

11. Persistent aches or pains, headaches, cramps, or digestive problems that don't ease with treatment.

Depression is stressful. The physical effects of chronic stress, added to poor self-care brought on by changes in energy levels, sleep, and appetite, can cause a variety of health problems.

What to look for: Increased self-medication (using, for example, pain relievers, alcohol, prescription meds, or illegal drugs, increased complaints that don't seem to fit any kind of pattern, increased doctor visits or refusal to see a doctor despite obvious complaints.

What else to know: Obviously any of these physical signs can be clues to health problems that are unrelated to depression. The point is to notice if these behaviors are clustering with other symptoms of depression — and to get them addressed by a health professional so that, whatever their origin, they become one (or two, or three, or five) fewer bothersome aspects of the depressed person's life.

Silver lining: Getting a loved one, or yourself, to a doctor to evaluate chronic symptoms allows you to also report the worrisome depressive symptoms, and get them checked out and, if necessary, treated. This is valuable, given that so many people with depression are in denial or reluctant to seek help. It's not a sign of weakness to be overwhelmed by caregiving!

Even better, the majority of cases of depression, even the most severe, respond to treatment, according to the National Institute of Mental Health.

o o o

More Sources of Help

I can't say it enough: You need all the help you can find. Whether you're just starting down the path of dealing with dementia, or deep into Alzheimer's care, don't miss the following resources:

Your local Area Agency on Aging (AAA)

What it is: Your local area agency on aging (AAA) is a government-mandated clearinghouse for general information about community eldercare services. These agencies also offer free referrals to local services that provide transportation, meals, adult day services, in-home caregivers, legal assistance, home-based training programs for caregivers, and other forms of help.

The names of these agencies often vary by community. But the services they refer to are usually free or low-cost, and calling the agency is free.

How it can help you: Area agencies on aging are one of the best first calls a caregiver can make to learn the local lay of the land on eldercare: what kinds of programs, facilities, and expertise are available in the community. This includes respite care, nutrition and transportation programs, home health services, legal services, housing options, and much more. Staffers can answer common questions and refer you to resources that are most likely to match your family's specific needs — speeding your research process and perhaps making you aware of resources you never knew existed.

To find: Start at www.n4A.org. (The "4" refers to the fourth A, as this is the website for the Association of Area Agencies on Aging.) You'll find a listing of local agencies to work from.

The Alzheimer's Association

What it is: Founded in 1980 as the first national organization devoted to advancing Alzheimer's disease awareness and research, the Alzheimer's Association now has more than 75 chapters and runs more than 4,500 local support groups. The organization also conducts extensive research fundraising.

How it can help you: Local chapters are one of the greatest assets to family caregivers, a handy way to tap into support groups and educational programs or connect with local experts. The Alzheimer's Association has also partnered with MedicAlert to provide a 24-hour emergency response service for medical emergencies or to find those who wander off. Another service, called Comfort Zone, lets families remotely monitor someone with Alzheimer's through automated alerts.

To find: Start at www.alz.org.

Local dementia support groups

What they are: Support groups come in many formats, but most involve small groups of people sharing common experiences under the guidance of a trained expert (such as a social worker or nurse) or a fellow caregiver. They're often held at hospitals, community centers, and places of worship. Participants meet at regular intervals to hear speakers, learn about local resources, and exchange practical ideas and emotional support.

Some groups target spouses or those dealing with a specific stage of dementia. There are also groups for the newly diagnosed, which may be run by hospitals or memory clinics, organizations such as the local Alzheimer's Association, social-services agencies, or self-starting individuals who are reaching out to fellow caregivers.

How they can help you: Participating in a support group outside of the home helps caregivers feel less isolated (a common complaint) both physically and emotionally. Others who are going through the same experiences share their stories, mistakes, and successes; strong friendships often form. Groups may feature expert speakers who discuss such relevant concerns as neuroscience, behavioral issues, Medicare, self-care, or family dynamics.

Research shows that participants in caregiver support groups report less stress and depression, and they may be better able to delay institutionalization of a loved one.

To find: Ask your loved one's doctor for recommendations. Also check community hospitals and local memory clinics or senior centers. Sometimes by starting with the local Alzheimer's Association chapter, you can learn about adjunct groups run by other organizations.

The Alzheimer's Disease Education and Referral Center (ADEAR)

What it is: Run by the National Institute on Aging, ADEAR is the government's consumer information center about Alzheimer's disease. ADEAR provides research summaries, free publications on memory loss and caregiving in English and Spanish, and general information about Alzheimer's disease.

ADEAR also manages National Institute on Aging-funded Alzheimer's Disease Centers, which are research centers at major medical institutions across the country. In addition, ADEAR manages the Alzheimer's Disease Clinical Trials Database, a joint program of the U.S. Food and Drug Administration and the National Institute on Aging.

How it can help you: The ADEAR's Alzheimer's Disease Centers can be good starting places for creating an action plan to cope with memory loss, especially if you live near one. They may offer diagnosis and medical management as well as access to clinical trials of dementia drugs. Participants in clinical trials usually receive free treatment and follow-ups in exchange for helping to advance drug research to slow or cure the disease.

To find: Start at www.nih.gov/alzheimers. Your doctor will be able to tell you if there's an Alzheimer's Disease Center near you. (They tend to be university-based.)

The Beers Criteria

What it is: Officially known as the Beers Criteria for Potentially Inappropriate Medication Use in Older Adults, this reference lists of more than 50 medications or classes of medications that carry potential risks for people over 65. It was updated in 2012 by a panel of experts in geriatrics. The list was created to help doctors, but anyone can use it.

How it can help you: If your loved one is prescribed a new medication or you're uncertain about his or her existing drug list, you want to check foremost with the doctor, of course. But if you have any questions, especially if the regular doctor is not a geriatrician, the Beers Criteria is worth a quick check for potential red flags. Listed, for example, are drugs that have a high risk of side effects or limited effectiveness (and better alternatives); medications for common problems that may actually worsen the disorder; and drugs that are best used with caution and careful monitoring.

To find: The American Geriatrics Society offers a PDF of a handy, printable card of these drugs; go to americangeriatrics.org and search "Beers."

The Family Caregiver Alliance (FCA)

What it is: The leading nonprofit organization supporting long-term family caregivers of all kinds (those caring for anyone from ill children to elders), the Family Caregiver Alliance focuses on education, services, research, and advocacy. Much of what FCA does is "behind the scenes" to the average caregiver: advocating for caregiver-friendly policies, conducting and promoting influential research, working with corporate human-resources officers, and advancing the profile of the growing army of unpaid family caregivers. But the organization also offers many practical services.

How it can help you: FCA's National Center on Caregiving offers tip sheets on such topics as family meetings and end-of-life choices. A resource called Family Care Navigator helps users locate publicly funded caregiver support programs in all 50 states. It also conducts caregiver workshops and professional training around the country.

To find: www.caregiver.org

Online support groups for caregivers

What they are: A digital twist on the conventional face-to-face support group, online support or chat groups provide the same kind of emotional understanding and practical advice-sharing. Some online support groups require enrolling as a member, while others are open to the general public. Most are sponsored by organizations or companies and are monitored.

How they can help you: Connecting with other caregivers in the same boat provides an outlet to vent when needed — no saving up tales of woe for, say, Thursdays at 7 p.m. You can also get the benefit of "group think" — hundreds or thousands of fellow caregivers share their answers and tips. Unlike conventional groups, you can get help right when you need it, even if it's 2 a.m. And because participants don't have to leave home, these groups are often a more practical option for those grappling with a loved one's moderate- to severe-stage dementia.

To find: Look at websites specializing in Alzheimer's care or caregiving. Caring.com, for example, provides stage-based community groups for those who use its "Steps & Stages" resource. (www.caring.com)

The Alzheimer's Store

What it is: An online shopping resource filled with products designed for people with Alzheimer's or other dementias, or that assist their caregivers. Many different stores and sites sell useful products, but this resource is worth being aware of because you can scan all sorts of items in one place.

How it can help you: Find hard-to-remove clothing, activities, safety items, easy-to-read clocks, and much more. It's also organized by stage.

To find: www.alzstore.com

Caring.com Steps & Stages

What it is: This first-of-its-kind, customizable, online resource for Alzheimer's care walks family members through everything they'll encounter while coping with a loved one's disease, including both expert guidance and support from fellow caregivers. Users answer a few basic questions to determine which stage of dementia-care advice they probably need. Then they receive weekly e-newsletters tailored to the common concerns of that stage, gain access to stage-specific discussion groups, receive critical self-care advice, and can ask experts questions or access a huge library of practical caregiving advice.

(Full disclosure: I was part of the team that developed "Steps & Stages.")

How it can help you: Because Alzheimer's is a progressive disease that's different for everyone, finding the specific help you need at a particular time can be overwhelming. The stage-based nature of Steps & Stages simplifies the challenge by tailoring advice to your loved one's condition right now.

To find: www.caring.com/steps-stages/alzheimer's

o o o

ACKNOWLEDGMENTS

I love writing lists like this, so I can give credit where it's truly due. At the same time, I hate such lists because I invariably leave off someone I should have included.

I regret, for example, not jotting down the names of everyone who shared a story or an insight with me, over the past six years I've spent writing about aging and Alzheimer's — at conferences and talks, in interviews for articles, in chat groups online and while anonymously exchanging "hugs and prayers" via Caring.com. I learned so much from my brief encounters with all of them.

Special thanks go to the many aging, caregiving, and dementia experts who inform my work. In the topmost tier, incalculably generous with their time and insights, have been Dr. Leslie Kernisan, Dr. Ken Robbins, and Duke University's Lisa Gwyther.

I'm also grateful to these stand-outs whom I've interviewed or come to know over the years: Dr. Richard Isaacson, Leeza Gibbons, Teepa Snow, Naomi Feil, Bob DeMarco, Amy Goyer, Barbara Kate Repa, Carol D. O'Dell, David Troxel, Joe Matthews, Ann Basting, Joyce Simard, Dr. Gary Small, Mark Warner, Ellen Warner, Geri Hall, Ann Cason, Beth Spencer, Joanne Koenig Coste, Neil Buckholtz, I-Fen Lin, Gail Hunt, Dr. Anton Porsteinsson, Dr. John Morris, Rhonda Montgomery, Dr. Vicki Rackner, Andrea Seewald, Jina Lewallen, Helene Bergman, Suzanne Mogliadini, Linda Fodrini-Johnson, Margit Novack, Dr. Eva Selhub, Steve Sultanoff, Dave Givens, Jamie Comstock, Guy Eakin, Robert Neimeyer, Maggie Callanan, Dr. Ira Byock, Linda Harootyan, Todd Kluss, and Kim Linder — and I know that's a too-short list.

Among my favorite "real life" experts and sounding boards on caregiving, I count Laura Patyk, Paul Patyk, Mary Gamble, Patti Anderson, Beth Hanes, Gary Joseph LeBlanc, Kay Strom, Brenda Avadian, Susan Morris, Mary Carter, Frank Winckowski, Amy Keller, Rhonda Swink, Jamie Blackmon, Santa Bogdon, Jamie Gannon, Camille Peri, and Bob Rachlow.

On an organizational level, Caring.com immersed me in this material and changed the direction of my life (more about that in a moment), so thank you, founder and CEO Andy Cohen. I've also been helped often along the way by Caring's Denise Graab and Shoghig Balkian.

Other helpful groups that contributed to this project include the Gerontological Society of America and New America Media, which together administer the Met Life Foundation Journalists in Aging fellowships; the National Press Foundation and its Alzheimer's Disease Issues journalist training program; the Journalists Network on Generations (and its tireless creator Paul Kleyman), the Family Caregiver Alliance, the Rosalynn Carter Institute for Caregiving, the Alzheimer's Foundation of America, and the Alzheimer's Association.

I also want to thank Megan Kempston, who acted as hands-on caregiver to the publishing process, and Allyson Appen for her helpful design advice.

Not last or least to be acknowledged — more like first and foremost — is Jim Scott. We got to know each other again, after a nearly 20-year silence, when he hired me to work for Caring.com, which he'd co-founded. A few years later, we married — and without his merciless nagging (I mean tireless loving encouragement and editorial savvy), I might never have finally collected my personal and professional experiences with dementia into *Surviving Alzheimer's*.

Thank you all.

o o o

ABOUT THE AUTHOR

PAULA SPENCER SCOTT has written extensively about Alzheimer's and other dementias. As a senior editor (now contributing editor) of the eldercare website Caring.com, she created its Alzheimer's channel, including its first-of-a-kind "Steps and Stages" Alzheimer's resource for family caregivers and related blogs. She's a fellow of both the Met Life Foundation Journalists in Aging Program and the National Press Foundation's Alzheimer's Disease Issues 2012. Active in caregiver education and research projects, she's been a presenter at Aging in America as well as "Conversations in Caregiving" webcasts for AlzheimersDisease.com. Four family members, including her late father, had dementia.

Scott is the author of 11 other books on health and family life, including *Momfidence* (based on her longtime Woman's Day magazine column), *Pregnancy Journal*, and the collaborations *The V Book*, *Bright From the Start*, and the New York Times bestseller *The Happiest Toddler on the Block*. She lives in the San Francisco Bay Area with her husband; they have six children.

You can find more information at her websites, survivingalzheimersbook.com and paulaspencerscott.com. Follow her on Twitter @PSpencerScott.

74593111R00204

Made in the USA
Lexington, KY
16 December 2017